Being Empathic

A companion for counsellors and therapists

Steve Vincent
Client-centred therapist
Person-centred supervisor, trainer and academic

Forewords by

Gay Leah Barfield

and

Veniamin Kolpachnikov

CRC Press
Taylor & Francis Group
Boca Raton London New York

CRC Press is an imprint of the
Taylor & Francis Group, an **informa** business

T0251843

Contents

Foreword

Reading this important new book has helped me note how far afield and adrift I have gone from practising as a person-centred therapist who once held complete trust in the core principles as being truly necessary and sufficient in themselves for therapy to be successful. As a result it helped me to return 'home' again with more trust in myself and the client.

Let's see what a 'cornucopia' of offerings are provided in this book, since this important exploration of Carl Rogers' work is about so much more than empathy, covering in fact nearly all the major constructs and concepts of Rogers' work during his lifetime.

Throughout this book, to support his subtle analyses of the principle of empathy in particular, Steve Vincent uses original source material faithfully, including impeccable research going as far back as 1937, to seek Carl's earliest conceptualisations. Steve has also minutely delved the depths of the major 1959 theoretical and scientific analysis by Carl of his own theory, using quotes from it throughout the work, thus both enlarging upon and deepening our understanding of the principles. If the reader were never to read these source works of Carl's in their entirety, then this book would provide beautifully clear explications of them.

The quotes and extracts from Rogers are always to the point, and explorations of the concepts rich and original, each amplifying, yet not changing, Carl's meanings. Steve also reminds us of some of Rogers' own seminal thinking that has perhaps been lost over the years; for example, citing an early quote of Carl's that the 'process of change' is rather an existential state of 'changingness', a unique paradox that in itself helps both the practitioner and the client be comfortable with an ongoing state of evolving and emergent ways of being.

While the audience for this book might best be considered to be those in training as therapists, or students using the book as a university text, it will also be most helpful for practitioners who want to review and renew a deeper understanding of Rogers' approach after practising for so long that they may have forgotten or put aside the core principles. Potential clients, in seeking a safe haven for their deep explorations, may also profit greatly from this book as a guide in their search.

How does this book advance our thinking?

The depth of Steve's intellect is shown in his creative new contributions to the advancement of our thinking and the refinement of our practices. As a contribution to the literature, the author minutely dissects the complexity of the principle and practice of empathy to a level rarely achieved elsewhere, and of other concepts as well. In the latter case, for example, he makes very clear for the learner/reader/practitioner the distinction between the actualisation tendency and self-actualisation, and between actualisation and the formative tendency, constructs that so often get misused, confused and misunderstood.

He also makes an important distinction between, and provides a precise definition of, resistance and avoidance, arguing that these concepts are inconsistent with the person-centred approach (PCA). In addition, he makes it clear that Carl was adamant about the disservice to relationship emanating from the concept of transference. Steve also objects to such a concept because it separates, not connects, people rather than creating what I term a 'reciprocal multi-directional empathy' that emerges in all directions as therapy evolves, without interference from such conceptual frames of separation.

There are many non-traditional insights, emphases and ideas throughout this book, such as the fresh notion that unconditional positive regard is the highest level of 'confrontation' and congruence. The examples the author uses to support his points are moving and precise, such as the young boy cutting himself, who moves towards self-understanding with his therapist by respecting and accepting all perspectives of his inner 'configurations'. In the writing about the 'as if' quality of empathy, there is a fine example of what the best of being objective means, and its relationship to being empathic. There is a creative acronym (VALID) to help us remember the state of clients when they enter therapy, and subtle analyses of each 'condition' needed for successful therapy, be there 3, 6 or 12! Enumerating the five early premises with which Carl began to articulate his approach from 1961 onwards is very helpful. The author makes a brilliant 'circular' reverse summation, intertwined and non-linear in nature, that shows the complete tapestry of person-centred principles as they weave together as a whole cloth.

I appreciate Steve's idea of the community being defined as various configurations' of self/selves, expressed through different voices. His clarification of the use of that term by Dave Mearns, and sourced originally by Carl himself, is quite eye-opening. In each chapter the author invites us to ask ourselves intellectually profound questions with no simple answers, helping us to dig deeper into even more fertile soil for thinking through our values and beliefs. This book is thus a profusion of possibilities for us all.

I am particularly interested in language, and in those parts of the book which focus on use of language the reader discovers very original contributions and additions to the PCA dialogue. Steve defines words such as perception, awareness, symbolisation, etc., with great precision, as Carl seemed to use them.

I may disagree somewhat with the author in his critique of there being too much emphasis on the importance of language in skills training. He seems to contradict himself on occasion, acknowledging the importance of the right word for a client, and thus the therapist, yet in some instances discounting the importance of words, thus presenting an internal contradiction for the reader to resolve for themselves, or to live with as a dual truth and find their own path – very person-centred!

How is this book different from others on the same subject?

This book has a unique format and style, merging tradition with innovation and whimsy. In the middle of the book, we are suddenly presented with a personal dialogue with Steve and an interviewer, which changes the pace and rhythm of the book entirely. In fact this interview encapsulates what the book is all about.

The interview is both intellectually stimulating and very personal, including the 'I' voice so derided in academia, and which Carl himself initiated for the first time in academic writing. It is a very thorough interview, engaging and stylistically different from the rest of the book. Steve reminds me here of Brian Thorne and Carl himself in how very honest and forthcoming he is about himself. This gives a further order of credibility to the rest of book.

I was delighted with the wit, humour, play on words, catchy headings, and the like which Steve uses throughout the text, whether in his personal interview segment, or within the theoretical analyses, making the latter sparkle, and more human and understandable for the reader. Steve uses these lighter devices while at the same time asking the reader to be intellectually stretched by the demands of the book. For example, he has fun with clever yet profound sub-titles, such as 'Thou shalt not skill', and at the same time addresses the deeper issue of: once I am 'de-skilled', who am I as a therapist? This is a very important idea, as if only through emptying my self can I discover myself.

No matter what the writing style or rhythm, the nature of Steve's enquiry is evocative and thorough, while he also takes strong and clear stands, such as objecting to some current misunderstandings of the person-centred approach and certain aspects of eclecticism popular today.

What might have been Carl's view of this book?

While none of us can speak for Carl, my guess is that he would be delighted to see how profoundly Steve has dissected, in a loving, respectful and scientific way, Carl's lifetime of evolutionary thinking, honouring his own scientist in that sense. I trust that he would be particularly pleased with how Steve has minutely parsed Carl's major 1959 work, of which he himself often said he was most proud as a mathematical and scientific conceptualisation. Steve shows both what a profound thinker Carl was, as well as the profound thinker that Steve is. When compared with the reductionistic, stereotypic depiction of Rogers' work in so many previous texts outside the PCA community, this book is a breath of fresh air.

The future

I would like to end this foreword with a particular emphasis on the values of love, spirituality and peace building, which, while not elaborated upon in particular by Steve in this text, seem to permeate this entire work and make it clear that, in fact, Carl's approach has always expressed these values. Although through no intention of the author, this book has thus deepened my own belief that this theory and its core concepts, particularly empathy, are readily transferable to other arenas beyond individual therapy, such as the larger social conflicts and crises wounding our suffering planet. Unfortunately some 43 years later, with a world in turmoil, Carl's 1961 quote below is still applicable. Perhaps it is our role to be the current catalysts to such realisation of these principles both inside the therapy office and for the larger public good.

> *Our civilization does not yet have enough faith in the social sciences to utilize their findings.*
>
> (Rogers 1961: p. 335)

In the closing years of his life, Carl made even more explicit his sense of the importance of love in our work, and his ever-present concern for the need for balance between the individual's self-concerns with an acknowledgement of our inevitable connectedness to each other. In the poignant quote below, published in 2002, he belies those critics who had long discounted or misunderstood the place of relationship in his philosophy by labelling it as narcissistic and hyper-individualistic.

> *in becoming more aware of self and others, in becoming more acceptant of self and others, and in becoming more understanding of self and others, people become more able to meaningfully live their lives, more . . . able to love, able to receive love.*
>
> (Rogers and Russell 2002: p. 258)

In this re-discovery of the richness of Rogers' approach that Steve has created for us by writing this book, he has guided us with elegance, insight, wisdom and compassion towards a deeper understanding of the genius and profundity of Carl Rogers' work and principles. For that reason, I look forward with enthusiasm and anticipation to his next books on the other core conditions, genuineness and unconditional positive regard.

Gay Leah Barfield PhD, MFT
Former Co-Director
Carl Rogers Institute for Peace
December 2004

Foreword

A step towards a better world

Every human being strives to live a life that brings them satisfaction and happiness. We search for ways to live such a life in an outer world, and that is not an easy enterprise.

Each race imbues in its members the ways and means of being that have been culturally and historically tested by the experience of previous generations. This take place through childbearing in families, through the process of education, through peer exchange of experiences, and in many other ways.

This process of providing culturally tested ways of being in the world is of great value and provides the essence of each person to become Human. Yet, it often imposes on a person ways and means of being (norms, values, ideas and ways of acting) that are inconsistent with the person's deepest and authentic strivings and intentions. The person starts to live an imposed life. This may be convenient, yet it does not bring deep satisfaction and happiness to that person, and the World (society, culture) is denied the full potential of that person's input, energy and creativity. Both the person and the World lose out.

In this book Steve Vincent deeply and carefully explores Empathy as a way of facilitating personal growth and being. It considers the way a person is able to become fully Themself in the World, bringing deep satisfaction and happiness to that person, and their full potential of energy, creativity and productivity to the World. (I am far from believing that the way is not without troubles and difficulties, but I do believe that this is the way for achieving dynamic harmony of the Person, the World and the Person in the World!)

At a personal and professional level, Steve Vincent is a writer to trust on the subject of empathy. Empathy for Steve, as I know him, is not just a technique for professional psychological work. Empathy is for him a way of being with people. This personal and professional commitment to empathy makes Steve Vincent's exploration of empathy really deep and comprehensive. In a very personal yet accurate way he presents the history of the development of the concept and practice of empathy in psychotherapy. What is evident is the deep impression and influence that Carl Rogers, the founder of the Person-centered Approach and one of the most famous and influential psychologists of the 20th century, had on Steve.

Throughout this book, the author – as scientist, professional psychotherapist and inquiring person – carefully and accurately presents his view on empathy in psychotherapy and interpersonal relationships. In Chapter 4, I value highly the systematic and convincing analysis made by Steve of the role and place of empathy in the process of facilitating personal growth. And I find very sincere and touching the self-Inter: View Steve makes in Chapter 3 as a way of exploring and expressing his personal notions of empathy.

The book is intended for professional psychologists and psychotherapists who look for ways of deeper understanding of, and ways of improving, their work with clients. The book will be invaluable for psychology students and interns who work on the understanding of human nature and on the development of their counseling style. But what is most valuable and inspiring for me is the way the book brings all of us closer to being ourselves, to enable one to be oneself with persons close to us – relatives, friends or clients – and to make the World we live in better!

Thank you, Steve, for your exquisite work!

Veniamin Kolpachnikov
Assistant Professor
Department of Psychological Counselling
Moscow City Psychology–Pedagogical University
Russia
December 2004

About the author

Steve Vincent, born in 1954, completed a sociology degree at the University of Sheffield, during which he was Chair and Trainer for Student Nightline. This was followed by a one-year full-time postgraduate Diploma in Counselling at the University of Aston in Birmingham. In 1999, at the University of East Anglia, he completed his Masters Degree, *On Becoming Person-Centred?* (Vincent 1999a) which involved researching the person-centred training of client-centred therapists.

Steve has worked as a youth counsellor in Liverpool (1980–82) and as a student counsellor in Southampton (1982–95), where he founded a person-centred training unit within a college of further education. After 21 years in further education, he resigned in an attempt to get a more person-centred life! He has been Membership Secretary, Chair and Newsletter Editor for BAPCA (British Association for the Person-Centred Approach) and is currently a BACP (British Association for Counselling and Psychotherapy) accredited practitioner as well as a Board member of CSP (Carl Rogers Center for Studies of the Person, La Jolla, California).

He now devotes most of his time to offering client-centred therapy in several GP practices, being a partner in a family and, from September 2002, a father for the first time. Carl Rogers, in reply to a question about the best way to make an organisation person-centred, said 'Start one' – so that's exactly what Steve did, and Client-Centred Therapy, Person-Centred Approach Services (CCTPCAS) was formed. It is now a project of CSP, and through it Steve and others offer a variety of person-centred events and activities in the UK.

You can contact Steve Vincent at cctpcas@aol.com or visit the CCTPCAS website at www.cctpcas.com, and you can find out more about CSP at www.centerfortheperson.org.

Introduction: the shape of this book

Prelude, substance and interlude

The primary purpose of this book is to provide a substantial text on empathic understanding – a kind of 'All you ever wanted to know about empathy, but were afraid you wouldn't find in one place' volume. As I reflected upon the development of my own understanding of, capacity for, experience and communication of empathy, two main factors stood out, namely learning about client-centred therapy (with reference to Carl Rogers in particular), and my own experiencing (which includes reflecting upon that experiencing). I wanted to somehow combine these two elements as both, it seemed to me, had validity and meaning. Furthermore, they have cross-fertilised and nourished each other over the years.

However, it seems that writing in the first person and from one's own experience is unacceptable to many publishers, who maintain that there are 'academic standards to uphold, reputations to consider', and so on. Yet mindful of Carl Rogers saying that what is most personal is most meaningful, I was delighted when researching some of the background for this book to come across the following:

> In the science of man, we are going to try to include emotions and affect, etc. Yet we operate on the absolute, unquestioned assumption that the best way of doing so will be somehow to put that in cognitive and intellectual terms . . . I can't but help wonder whether there may not some day be a new conception of science which would involve communication of more than intellectual symbols. . . . There may be ways of getting at knowledge and communicating knowledge which question the whole damn underlying assumption that science consists of nothing but symbols, all of which must necessarily be intellectual.
>
> (Rogers 1989: p. 164)

So, at one time, I tried to blend the academic and the experiential into the ongoing text. Up to a point this seemed to work well enough, yet beyond that point it began to feel a little fuzzy, a little unclear. Next I decided to leave all of my personal musings out altogether, yet this felt like unwelcome censorship, whether undertaken by myself or by a would-be publisher. Then, finally, I hit on the idea of 'interludes' – interspersing the core journey, derived overwhelmingly from the work of Carl Rogers, with sightseeing trips of my own, derived from my experience. Several more personal (and hence meaningful, at least to me) articles were earmarked for inclusion as interludes, among them *On Becoming More Whole? Necking in Glasgow* (Vincent 1999b), *A Training Trip Through Empathy* (Vincent 1999c), *From Whole to Hole to Whole* (Vincent 2000a), *Failing or Fortunate? Striving for Revising* (Vincent 2000b), *Setting Aside or Erupting?* (Vincent 2001), *Client-Centred Therapy: Conditions, Process and Theory* (Vincent 2002a), *Empathy: an inter-view* (Vincent 2002b) and a few poems. It transpired that the inclusion of these as interludes would have taken the word count of this book way beyond the optimum publishing size, so while *Empathising in action: an inter-view* has been retained as Chapter 3 of this book (in the belief that it serves to bring together many of the emergent threads up to that point and to pave the way for some of what follows, all in a less formal fashion), all of the others are omitted (the omitted articles are available via the CCTPCAS website at www.cctpcas.com).

I have tried to use gender-free terminology in my own writing. Quotes from Carl Rogers (of which there are many) tend to be couched in masculine form, and these are given verbatim. In his later years, Carl apologised for this, writing, for example:

> I regret that in this paper, written some years ago, I used 'he' as the generic term. I hope my feminine readers will forgive me. I have learned better since.
>
> (Rogers 1986: pp. 2–3, 23)

Although some readers may care to skip my introductory comments, a 'prelude' is nevertheless provided in an attempt to offer a very basic 'level playing field' – a shared understanding from which the rest can follow.

I hope that it works for you.

Rogers; Carl; Carl Rogers; Rogers, Carl

In writing this book, I struggled somewhat in determining how to refer to Carl Ransom Rogers (1902–1987). In various drafts I tried only using *Carl*, only using *Rogers*, and using only *Carl Rogers*. Feedback from my 'critical friends' was divided. Some liked the use of *Carl*, as it had a kind of familiar, friendly, warm feeling to it. Others disliked this – for precisely the same reason (together with an opinion that it didn't come across as sufficiently 'academic'). This group tended to prefer the use of *Rogers*, yet the first group felt this to be impersonal and cold, even 'needlessly academically conventional'. The use of *Carl Rogers* (or even *Carl R Rogers*) all the time seemed even more formal, put the word count up, and frankly became somewhat tedious, even boring, yet clearly some critical friends preferred it this way. It seemed that whatever form of address I chose, one-third would be happy and two-thirds unhappy. Funnily enough, in all draft versions all 'proper' quoted *references* were to Rogers, Carl – no problem there! (And most of the references in this book *are* to Carl Rogers, Carl or Rogers – this is a book about client-centred empathy as a Carl Rogers companion.)

And what of my own feelings and thoughts? Well, I settled on a mix of all three forms of address. Often *Carl* somehow just 'felt right' and sometimes *Rogers* seemed more apt, while at other times *Carl Rogers* seemed to fit best. There were other times when there was little sense of 'rightness', so my choice was either based on varying the text or was random. 'Maybe', I ended up thinking, 'even if I certainly couldn't please *all* of the readers *all* of the time, I could at least please *some* of the readers *some* of the time'.

And you know I really don't think that Carl would have minded much one way or the other.

Client-centred therapy/person-centred approach

References throughout this book are, in the main, to *client-centred therapy*. The term *person-centred* is less frequently used. However, the words *counselling* and *therapy* are used interchangeably (consistent with Carl Rogers who also treated these words as being synonymous). Carl wrote and spoke many times of the changes in terminology that were introduced over the years – for example, as applications drawn from therapy became more and more diverse:

> As client-centered therapy became applied in the field of education, it wasn't therapy, so what was it? Student-centered education? Gradually it became quite evident that we weren't talking about therapy in these other fields, so what was it? That was when we began to adopt the term *person-centered*, which still implies a lot of reliance on the internal frame of reference, but it's not therapy.
>
> (Rogers and Russell 2002: p. 253)

Debates over what is client-centred and what is person-centred (or indeed whether the two are one and the same thing) abound, it seems. Although I have my own views, I'd like Carl to have the last (or even the definitive) word on this. Just prior to his death in February 1987, he wrote that wrangling over the differences between these two terms was futile, as he, Carl Rogers, was the *same person*, with access to the same personal resources, whether he was meeting a client for one-to-one therapy or facilitating a large group. Historically, the term *person-centred approach* arose from a need to encompass the many diverse applications of the philosophy, theory and practices that grew out of the learning gathered from *client-centred*, one-to-one therapy – *activities* such as trainee-centred learning, encounter groups, relationships (including parenting), conflict transformation, and so on. Rogers conceded that a label for this diversity could well be more open to loose use, misuse and misunderstanding, yet he stated that nevertheless he 'would like a term to describe what I do when I am endeavoring to be facilitative in a group of persons who are *not* my clients', and that term was *person-centred* (Rogers 1987a: p. 12).

To me, this couldn't be more clear. One-to-one counselling is client-centred therapy, whereas non-client-work activities based on the principles that arose from client-centred therapy constitute a person-centred approach. The facilitative and/or therapeutic *person* may well be the same (or very similar) in both, but the *activity* is different. Nonetheless, as the bulk of Carl's writing about empathy is in the context of client-centred therapy, that term takes precedence in this book.

Client-centred therapy: core/necessary and sufficient conditions

What a horrible word *conditions* is in some respects! The word 'respects' in this context brings to mind the word *respect* in another context – that is, linked with *unconditional* positive regard. How strange it seems to have *unconditional* as part of a *condition*!

Over the years, Carl Rogers penned several versions of 'conditions' – for therapy, for personality change, for trainee-centred learning, for facilitative group leadership, and so on. In 1942, for example, there were four conditions, namely *objectivity, respect for the individual, understanding of the self* and *psychological knowledge* (*see* Chapter 1). At other times, there have been four quite different *necessary and sufficient* conditions, or five, or six – or there are what have become known as the three *core* or *therapist* conditions, namely congruence, unconditional positive regard and empathic understanding, although even the wording of these changed over time. For instance, what was first known as *acceptance* in the early days of client-centred therapy later came to be known as *unconditional positive regard*. Some people erroneously believe that Rogers planned to introduce a *seventh* condition of intuition, or an *eighth* condition of spirituality. Their belief is erroneous because Carl saw intuition as part of empathic understanding, and a 'spiritual' (although he was wary of this word) or 'transcendental' connection as part of both unconditional positive regard and empathy.

And so on. No doubt the debates will continue.

For the purposes of this book, the central version referred to is Carl's *Conditions of the Therapeutic Process* (Rogers 1959), otherwise known as the six necessary and sufficient conditions for therapeutic personality change, as described below.

For therapy to occur it is necessary that the following conditions exist.

1   Two persons are in *contact*.
2   The first person, whom we shall term the client, is in a state of *incongruence*, being *vulnerable* or *anxious*.
3   The second person, whom we shall term the therapist, is *congruent* in the relationship.
4   The therapist is *experiencing unconditional positive regard* toward the client.
5   The therapist is *experiencing* an *empathic* understanding of the client's *internal frame of reference*.
6   The client *perceives*, at least to a minimal degree, conditions 4 and 5, the *unconditional positive regard* of the therapist for him, and the *empathic* understanding of the therapist (Rogers 1959: p. 213).

At times, Carl referred to condition 1 as a *pre*-condition, leaving five 'main' conditions. At other times, he wrote that conditions 1 and 2 could be considered as pre-conditions, leaving four 'main' conditions, three of which had been termed 'core' conditions, and so on. Academically or historically interesting as it may be to wrangle over just how many 'conditions' there are (or indeed over which is the 'correct' or 'definitive' version), what I would personally prefer is to distil and preserve the *essence* of the spirit of client-centred principles, attitudes and beliefs as I believe Carl Rogers intended them.

Before the beginning . . .

First and foremost, let us not forget throughout this exploration that empathy, or empathic understanding, is but one of the conditions for therapeutic personality change. When Carl Rogers and his colleagues researched what seemed to be effective and meaningful in therapeutic encounters, certain threads were identified as integral parts of the whole experience. While it is possible (and perhaps necessary) to examine each strand of this rich weave as a discrete aspect of client-centred therapy, it is helpful to remember that each necessary and sufficient strand remains a *part* of a *whole* – to remember to put back together the entire fabric once we have examined a weft, weave or thread. Alternatively, while it might be desirable to carve up the meal that is client-centred therapy into bite-sized chunks, let us not lose sight of the entire dish. In illustration of this point, Carl's daughter Natalie wrote:

> I remember one discussion group, however, that has stayed in my mind and heart. A large group of person-centered folks (including Carl) were sitting in a circle. The topic turned to 'Is it client-centered to do this, or client-centered to do that?'. There were disagreements, and case samples focusing on the minutiae of what a therapist said or did, with criticisms of this or that wording or behavior. My guts were tight, my breathing tense. I looked across the circle at Carl and his shoulders were slumped, his eyes focused on the floor. My unspoken thoughts were: 'Is the person-centered approach going to self-destruct by nit-picking every word a therapist says and losing sight of the essence of the I–thou relationship? Are we focusing on the precise verbalisations while losing the vision of being in tune with the client? Do we really know how to be a companion with the client on her road to self-discovery?'. I was angry and disappointed at the level of the discussion. Then Carl spoke. He heaved a big sigh and said 'Boy, am I glad that when I discovered this process I didn't have to figure out "Is it client-centered or not?" I was really just looking to see what worked for the client.' My spirit rose and in my heart I said 'Right on, Dad!'.
>
> (Rogers N 1997: p. 271)

So perhaps we can keep in mind the essence of all that constitutes a client-centred whole as we explore that portion of it which is empathic understanding.

Prelude

This brief overview is included for two main reasons – in part to define some key concepts for readers new to client-centred therapy, and in part because even the understanding of those familiar with client-centred therapy often seems to vary (for example, those who have stated that they are unaware of any difference between the *actualising tendency* and *self-actualising*, or those who see no contradiction in delivering skills training).

Client-centred therapy: an overview

According to Carl Rogers, the most well known of the founders of client-centred therapy, this approach to counselling could be deemed to have begun in 1940:

> On December 11, 1940, before an invited audience at the University of Minnesota, he delivered a lecture entitled 'Newer Concepts in Psychotherapy', and he subsequently came to consider the date of this event as the birthday of client-centered therapy.
>
> (Thorne, cited in Rogers and Russell 2002: p. 11)

Not long before he died, Carl Rogers (writing in partnership with Nat Raskin) stated that client-centred therapy (and the person-centred approach) was:

> a clearly stated theory, accompanied by the introduction of verbatim transcriptions of psychotherapy, [that] stimulated a vast amount of research on a revolutionary hypothesis: that a self-directed growth process would follow the provision and reception of a particular kind of relationship characterised by genuineness, non-judgmental caring, and empathy.
>
> (Rogers and Raskin 1989: p. 155)

Rogers linked this self-directed growth process with the idea of an organic *actualising tendency*, believing that in parallel with a *formative tendency*, based on *syntropy* (an innate universal drive to grow and become more complex, as opposed to *entropy*, the decaying of matter), there is a fundamental and integral characteristic of humans, *given the right conditions*, to be constructive, cooperative, social, responsible beings. Talking about his 1942 publication *Counseling and Psychotherapy*, Rogers said:

> The central theme was the notion that the potential for better health resided in the client . . . So the counsellor endeavored to create an interpersonal situation in which material could come into awareness. [By 1950] There was a great deal of stress on both the philosophical and attitudinal characteristics of the therapist, and a definite move away from techniques with perhaps a bit of groping toward a close personal relationship.
>
> (Rogers and Evans 1975: p. 24)

Rogers wrote and spoke of his growing disillusionment with both his 'traditional' working practices and his theoretical training. At one stage he wrote:

> It is the client who knows what hurts, what directions to go, what problems are crucial, what problems have been deeply buried. It began to occur to me that unless I had a need to demonstrate my own cleverness and learning, I would do better to rely on the client for the direction of movement in the process.
>
> (Rogers 1961: p. 12)

A consequence of this dawning belief in the client being at the heart of therapy (the client's *internal frame of reference* – how the client sees their own world) was 'out with the old and in with the new' ways of being. Counsellors aligned with such beliefs began to refrain from advising, manipulating, directing, interpreting or teaching clients, as such directive practices were increasingly seen as either at best irrelevant, or at worst damaging with regard to clients accessing and utilising their own capacities. The primary aim became as follows:

> That the client should grow toward *himself*, not toward Freud, Jung, or Rogers, is the fundamental understanding of nondirectiveness. To advise him how to behave, what to do, what to think, or how to act is a violation of the priority of his own phenomenal world.
>
> (Barton 1974: p. 180)

Thus in its origins what became known as client-centred therapy began as a reaction against traditional therapist attitudes and behaviours:

> There is no doubt that the term *nondirective* was in itself accurate, but it was a term of rebellion. It was saying what we were against. We were opposed to the highly directive kind of procedures being used. Then, as we became more secure, I think, in the fact that this was a new way, a legitimate way of proceeding, we began to recognize that it was centered in the client's frame of reference – that what we were endeavoring to do was to get within the client and release what was there. It was centered in the client in a way that was quite specific and quite deep. That term is often misunderstood. A lot of people say, 'I'm centered in the client', meaning 'I pay a lot of attention to my client'. We meant something deeper than that. Really this was built around the client's internal frame of reference, his inner world.
>
> (Rogers and Russell 2002: p. 253)

Carl Rogers was a leading pioneer in developing a more 'humanistic' approach to psychotherapy. However, learning derived from therapy began to be applied in increasingly diverse areas, and likewise the terminology that was used to describe what was going on came to have increasingly diverse interpretations, too. Rogers wrote:

> I smile as I think of the various labels I have given to this theme during the course of my career – nondirective counselling, client-centred therapy, student-centred teaching, group-centred leadership. Because the fields of application have grown in number and variety, the label 'person-centred approach' seems the most descriptive.
>
> (Rogers 1981: pp. 114–15)

Patterson (and Watkins) wrote that:

> Rogers uses two terms: *client-centered therapy* and the *person-centered approach*. Later, in an article entitled 'Client-Centered? Person-Centered?' Rogers states he would like 'a term to describe what I do when I am endeavoring to be facilitative in a group of persons who are not my clients.' That term is *person-centered*. *Client-centered* is the term used with clients, in therapy.
>
> (Patterson and Watkins 1996: p. xv)

Perhaps the most comprehensive presentation of what client-centred therapy is all about (certainly according to Carl Rogers himself) was published in 1959. Carl said:

> I worked harder on this theoretical formulation than on anything I have written before or since. It is, in my estimation, the most rigorously stated theory of the process of change in personality and behavior which has yet been produced . . . I suspect these volumes are in fact very little used. Certainly my chapter 'A Theory of Therapy, Personality, and Interpersonal Relationships, as Developed in the Client-Centered Framework' is the most thoroughly ignored of anything I have written. This does not particularly distress me, because I believe theories too often become dogma, but it has, over the years, perplexed me.
>
> (Rogers and Evans 1975: pp. 135–6)

Drawing from this and other sources, we can try to achieve a brief overview of client-centred attitudes, beliefs, processes and outcomes. What is it all about? Rogers wrote:

> Psychotherapy deals primarily with the organization and the functioning of the self.
>
> (Rogers 1951: p. 40)

If 'dealing' with the self is a fundamental aspect of therapy, perhaps it might be helpful to know a little of what is meant by this. It is interesting that originally Rogers was not too concerned with the 'self' as:

> I certainly didn't start psychological work being interested in anything as vague as the self. To me, that seemed like old-fashioned introspectionism. I was really forced to examine self and forced to define it for myself, because my clients in therapy kept using that term in all kinds of significant ways.
>
> (Rogers and Evans 1975: p. 15)

In the client-centred personality theory that developed as a consequence of researching and exploring the notion of 'self,' it was stated that the forming of a *self-concept* (through which experience is perceived) follows basic human needs in infancy for *positive regard* from others (a need for love and affection, which when experienced result in feelings of warmth, liking, respect, sympathy and acceptance to and for the other person). This in turn generates needs for *positive self-regard* (a good feeling towards the self that is no longer dependent on the attitudes of others) – and all too often this results in the actualising tendency becoming thwarted by these *conditions of worth* (the positive or negative valuing of experiencing based on the values of others rather than whether the experiencing enhances or fails to enhance the person). Rogers had thought about and researched how clients entering therapy seemed to be, finally settling on the term *incongruence* as a description:

> It seemed to me that psychological maladjustment is the degree of discrepancy between the self as perceived and the experiences that are going on within the organism. In psychological adjustment there is a greater congruence between these two.
>
> (Rogers and Russell 2002: p. 251)

In other words, incongruence is a psychological process whereby experiences that are not consistent with a person's self-concept, or self-image, may be *denied* to awareness altogether – or the perception of such an experience may be 'twisted' to such an extent that the experience can be admitted to consciousness, but only in a *distorted* fashion. Feelings or sensations accompany these psychological processes:

> When the individual has no awareness of such incongruence in himself, then he is merely vulnerable to the possibility of anxiety and disorganization. . . . If the individual dimly perceives such an incongruence in himself, then a tension state occurs which is known as anxiety.
>
> (Rogers 1957a: p. 97)

Clients are likely to be *defensive* if their self-concept is *threatened* by experiencing, and they may feel *low self-esteem*. Thus they bring both their *incongruence* (including vulnerability, anxiety, tension, low self-esteem and psychological defensiveness) and their *potential* to therapy, where they come into contact with a person who holds genuineness, non-judgemental caring and empathy as fundamental 'core' conditions of being a counsellor. These therapist attitudes were renamed and modified over time, until eventually the terms *congruence, unconditional positive regard* and *empathic understanding* became the most generally accepted terminology. It is these core conditions that Rogers believed were both *necessary* and *sufficient* to 'interface' with the client's conditions of worth and to facilitate constructive change:

> The goal of therapy is fostered by the therapist through the providing of three conditions. . . . If they are sufficient, then no other conditions are necessary. The only means of influencing the client are through these conditions. Any other active intervention by the therapist is inconsistent with the basic assumption of the existence of the drive toward self-actualization. The three conditions offered by the therapist frees the operation of this drive in the client. The perception of these conditions by the client results in client self-disclosure, self-exploration, self-directed and self-discovery learning leading to changes in client perceptions and attitudes that result in changes in behavior. These changes are elements of the self-actualizing process. They are unique for each client (though there are some common elements).
>
> (Patterson 2000: p. 183)

Thus six client-centred conditions, considered as both necessary and sufficient, emerged as two people being in contact, the client being incongruent, the therapist being congruently respectful and empathic, and the client perceiving the therapist's unconditional positive regard and empathic understanding (*see* Introduction, page 4).

Although it is not known for sure, it seems likely that either Carl Whitaker or a colleague of his coined the term congruence, for in an interview in 1958, Rogers said 'I think I essentially picked up this idea from the Atlanta group that's working with Carl Whitaker' (Kirschenbaum 1979: p. 196). Carl Rogers defined *congruence*, or genuineness, as meaning:

> the psychotherapist is what he *is*, when in the relationship with his client he is genuine and without 'front' or facade, openly being the feelings and attitudes which at that moment are flowing in him . . . the feelings the therapist is experiencing are available to him, available to his awareness, and he is able to live these feelings, be them, and able to communicate them if appropriate.
>
> (Rogers 1961: p. 61)

A client-centred therapist attempts to experience unconditional positive regard for clients. Stanley Standal (a student studying with Rogers) was somewhat dissatisfied with the term 'acceptance' as being too open to different interpretations, so he coined the term *unconditional positive regard* as meaning a deep, respectful and genuine *unconditional* caring or 'prizing' of clients – 'unconditional' in the sense that the caring is not contaminated by evaluation or judgement of the client's feelings, thoughts and behaviour as good or bad (Standal 1954). Therapists value and warmly accept the client without placing stipulations on that acceptance.

> The therapist expresses this quality of genuine regard through *empathy*. Being empathic reflects an attitude of profound interest in the client's world of meanings and feelings as the client is willing to share this world. The therapist receives these communications and conveys appreciation and understanding, with the effect of encouraging the client to go further or deeper. An interaction occurs in which [the therapist] is a warm, sensitive, respectful companion in the typically difficult exploration of another's emotional world.
>
> (Rogers and Raskin 1989: p. 157)

Client-centred therapy: a summary

The acronym 'VALID' can be used to characterise clients entering therapy, in that they are likely to be:

Vulnerable and
Anxious, feeling
Low self-esteem or worth, being in a relative state of
Incongruence and
Defensive.

Ideally, it is hoped that upon commencing therapy, clients will engage with a therapist who will *be* congruent and from whom they will receive unconditional positive regard *for* them and empathic understanding *of* them. These *therapist conditions* interact with the *client's conditions* (of worth), thereby generating a therapeutic *process* within which change and growth can occur, primarily through clients 'rediscovering' the potential of their actualising tendency. However, as has so often been commented upon:

> Rogers has elaborated on most of these points many times. Yet there appear to be many who call themselves client-centered who seem to be unaware of their implications for practice. Such therapists appear to have little faith in the actualizing tendency in their clients.
> (Patterson 2000: p. 183)

Client-centredness is 'borne on the therapist's shoulders' (Barton 1974: p. 185), for if a therapeutic encounter is to be client-centred in nature, it is up to the *therapist* to initiate and maintain it:

> If I can provide a certain type of relationship, the other person will discover within himself the capacity to use that relationship for growth, and change and personal development will occur.
> (Rogers 1961: p. 33)

This process of growth flows through many stages or phases:

> With all his ambivalences, the client wants to grow, wants to mature, wants to face his problems and work them through. Accept and clarify his initial expressions of feeling, and a fuller, deeper expression of feelings will follow. Accept and clarify these and insight will spontaneously occur. Accept and clarify these insights, and the client will begin to take positive actions in his life, based on this insight. Accept and clarify the meaning the client sees in his positive actions, and at some point, when he feels enough self-acceptance, self-understanding, and confidence in his ability to continue to deal with his own problems, he will end the relationship.
> (Kirschenbaum 1979: p. 128)

Client-centred theory is, as Rogers put it, of the *'if–then'* variety, the first *if* being the therapist core conditions. *If* a therapist holds a belief and trust in the inner capacities of clients and is authentically respectful and understanding in contact with incongruent clients, *then* a therapeutic process will naturally follow. *If* a therapeutic relationship exists, characterised by a genuine counsellor accepting and empathically understanding clients as they unfold through this process, *then* predictable outcomes follow:

> The conditions we have chosen to establish predict such behavioral consequences as these: that the client will become self-directing, less rigid, more open to the evidence of his senses, better organized and integrated, more similar to the ideal which he has chosen for himself. . . . We have set the conditions which predict various classes of behavior – self-directing behaviors, sensitivity to realities within and without, flexible adaptiveness – which are by their very nature

unpredictable in their specifics . . . scientific progress has been made in identifying those conditions in an interpersonal relationship which, if they exist in *B*, are followed in *A* by greater maturity in behavior, less dependence on others, an increase in expressiveness as a person, an increase in variability, flexibility, and effectiveness of adaptation, an increase in self-responsibility and self-direction . . .

(Rogers and Evans 1975: pp. lxxvi–vii)

In other words, while the outcomes of therapy are *predictable*, what can be predicted is the *unpredictable*, because clients grow towards actualising the unique and rich, complex and ever-changing individual potential that resides within all human beings.

Empathic understanding: origins and developments

In the beginning, there was the word

Dictionary corner . . .

. . . and the word was *empathy*. The *Concise Oxford Dictionary* defines empathy as the:

> Power of identifying oneself mentally with (and so fully comprehending) a person or object of contemplation.

Derived initially from the Greek 'empiateia' (meaning 'passionate affection') and later from the German language, current usage of the word *empathy* comes from the German words *ein* meaning 'in' and *fuhlung* meaning 'feeling' (from the Greek *pathos*, literally meaning 'suffering', also related to the Greek *penthos*, meaning 'grief'). Thus we could elaborate by saying that empathy means the power of projecting your own personality into, fully comprehending and being *in-feeling* with another – possibly with their suffering or grief. The *Concise Oxford Dictionary* also refers us to the word *sympathy*, which is defined as a '(capacity for) being simultaneously affected with the same feeling as another; tendency to share or state of sharing another person's emotion or sensation or condition; mental participation *with* another in his trouble or *with* another's trouble; compassion or approval (*for*); agreement (*with*) in opinion or desire', and the word *sympathetic* is defined as 'touches the feelings by association, etc.'. The meaning of the prefix *sym* is derived from 'alike' or 'as'.

Comparing *empathy* and *sympathy* might be helpful. Despite the italicising of 'with' in the definitions of sympathy, most common usage of the word would seem to be about feeling sympathy *for* or *towards* another, rather than 'projecting' *into* the feelings of another. Empathy might be likened to *insight* into the feelings of another ('This is how you feel . . .'), as compared with a sympathetic *associating with* or *feeling alike* ('I know just how you feel . . .'), or indeed questioning ('How do you feel . . .?'). In the definitions of *sympathy* appear the words *'approval for'* and *'agreement with'*, which again might help us to differentiate. *Empathy* is not to do with agreement or approval, but rather it is to do with insight into the feelings of another – *without judgement*.

Then there was Carl Rogers

Just one of several possible ways into an exploration of empathy is to chart the history of this therapeutic condition with reference to developments in client-centred thinking and practice. To this end, 'snapshots' have been selected from near the beginning, somewhere around the middle, and near the end of the career of Carl Ransom Rogers (1902–1987). So what follows is selective, for while researching this chapter it became abundantly clear that charting the historical development of empathy in the writings of Rogers could not be undertaken adequately without significant reference to other contextual elements – and especially to what were to become known as the *core conditions* (of congruence, unconditional positive regard and empathic understanding), and indeed to all six of the necessary and sufficient conditions for therapeutic personality change. Nevertheless, the snapshot references that follow were chosen with a primary focus on empathy – after all, this is a book about empathy!

Later in his life (in 1986), Carl Rogers was asked (by David Russell) to recall his first ever experience of empathy. Carl had vivid memories of being interviewed for a sexual issues survey by Dr Gilbert Van Tassel Hamilton. Rogers said that up until that moment in the 1930s:

> I think I had learned how to go more deeply into social interchange with friends, but as far as being really, thoroughly, deeply listened to, I don't know that that had been a part of my experience.
> (Rogers and Russell 2002: pp. 97–8)

Through being interviewed by Dr Hamilton, Carl Rogers realised all kinds of things about the self-expression of 'hidden' subject matter and how risky it can be to both say things and be heard. He also learned, through 'being on the receiving end', something about how someone might really listen to another person.

Way back in 1942, Carl Rogers wrote in his book *Counseling and Psychotherapy* that the *four* necessary qualifications to practise counselling were *objectivity, respect for the individual*, an *understanding of the self* and *psychological knowledge* (Rogers 1942: pp. 253–6). *Objectivity*? Students of client-centred therapy, especially those more familiar with modern thinking and practice, might feel somewhat surprised that the very first condition identified by Carl Rogers was *objectivity*, as it has a somewhat cold, dispassionate, disengaged feel to it. However, even in the early days of Carl's work we can see the origins of what was to come. For instance, he wrote:

> There are certain personal qualities which should be present if the individual is to develop into a good counselor, but there is no reason to believe that these are any more rare than the qualities which would be necessary for a good artist or a first-class aviation pilot. This is definitely true if we are talking of the client-centered type of counseling.
> (Rogers 1942: p. 253)

Here, then, is a message of hope for the would-be therapist. Even in 1942 Carl Rogers was saying that *being a person* was a primary requisite for counsellors – that therapists are not a 'class apart' from others. However, Rogers did write somewhat scathingly of 'directive' counsellors, stating that even in recorded interviews directive counsellors opined with some assurance on issues as diverse as the philosophy of life, racial prejudice, history, parents, marriage, vocational choice, discipline and:

> in fact, all the puzzling personal questions which a perplexed individual can face. The directive counselor, to be sure, has need of more omnipotent qualities . . . obviously a generous portion of supernatural wisdom is required of the individual who takes such an attitude toward counseling.
>
> (Rogers 1942: p. 253)

Rogers proposed a more modest aim for client-centred counselling, namely, to free individuals in order that they might utilise their own capacities and resolve issues for themselves. Within this context, he believed that a prerequisite for counsellors was that they would be 'sensitive to human relationships', and he wrote of awareness and 'social sensitivity' – sensing and being alert to subtle differences – and of these qualities combining to form a solid and natural foundation for the would-be therapist.

Objectivity

Having presented social sensitivity as a *pre*-condition, Rogers then identified *objectivity* as the first condition:

> It is generally conceded that to be helpful as a therapist the clinical worker needs to have an objective attitude. This has been variously described as 'controlled identification', as 'constructive composure', and as 'an emotionally detached attitude'.
>
> (Rogers 1939: p. 281)

This, as stated above, was back in 1939 – and it would seem to bear little relation to what we now understand as empathic understanding. Yet the seeds of what was to grow into the fifth necessary and sufficient condition for client-centred therapy were evident. Perhaps just as Carl remarked upon the actualising tendency being akin to tuber tendrils seeking the light in a darkened environment, so an analogy might be drawn from the words that followed, when he quoted himself:

> The term as used in clinical practice is defined somewhat differently. . . . There is included in the concept a capacity for sympathy which will not be overdone, a genuinely receptive and interested attitude, a deep understanding which will find it impossible to pass moral judgments or be shocked and horrified.
>
> (Rogers 1939: p. 283)

So in a sense, although Rogers used the word 'objectivity', he seemed to be somehow refining or redefining its everyday definition, stressing that this objectivity was neither a 'cold and impersonal detachment' nor 'deeply sympathetic and sentimental'. He also stated that the client-centred counsellor does not become so immersed in the world of the client as to be unable to enable that client. There is, he wrote:

> a degree of sympathetic 'identification' . . . sufficient to bring about an understanding of the feelings and problems . . . but an identification which is 'controlled', because understood, by the therapist.
>
> (Rogers 1939: p. 283)

Might we be able to see herein the origins of what Rogers later described as the 'as if' quality of empathic understanding – entering a client's world of feelings and meanings as if it were your own, yet without ever losing the *as if* quality? Just as empathic understanding is now seen as the fifth of the six necessary and sufficient conditions, so in 1942 *objectivity* was set within the context of other conditions, which were *respect for the individual, self-understanding* and *psychological knowledge*.

Respect for the individual

Carl wrote that *respect for the individual* meant a 'deep-seated respect' for the integrity of the client. The zealous, reforming therapist, who seeks to mould clients in the image of the counsellor, would be unable to establish a growth-promoting relationship with clients. *Acceptance of clients as they are*, and permitting clients the freedom to discover their own personal solutions, were seen as the key factors in respecting the individual. Here we can see the beginnings of what would later become known as *unconditional positive regard*.

Self-understanding

An *understanding of the self* included self-knowledge in terms of 'emotional patterns, and . . . limitations and shortcomings', for:

> Thoroughly to understand and be objective . . . the therapist must have some insight into his own personality.
>
> (Rogers 1939: p. 283)

Carl Rogers wrote of the necessity of personal insight in order to achieve an awareness of inner warps and biases due to personal feelings and prejudices, stressing the importance of supervision and counselling for therapists (the therapy being provided by the therapist's supervisor if necessary!). So here we can see the origins of what became known as *congruence*. It is perhaps interesting to note at this point that in 1942 Rogers placed objectivity *first*, whereas in later years empathic understanding became the *last* of the three therapist conditions. Yet even in these early days, there was a sense in which respect and self-understanding (later to become unconditional positive regard and congruence) were seen as necessary precursors to objectivity.

Psychological knowledge

Finally, Rogers wrote of *psychological knowledge*, stating that:

the therapist can scarcely expect to do satisfactory work without a thorough basis of knowledge of human behavior and of its physical, social and psychological determinants.

(Rogers 1939: p. 284)

Carl believed that many might expect psychological knowledge to be the *first* condition – yet stunning intellect was no guarantor of effective therapy:

The essential qualifications of the psychotherapist lie primarily . . . in the realm of attitudes, emotions and insight, rather than in the realm of intellectual equipment.

(Rogers 1939: p. 284)

Even earlier than this (in *Family* magazine in 1937), Carl had written of non-forcing, non-critical, accepting 'workers' who gave clients the fullest opportunity to grow.

Just four years on from the publication of his book entitled *Counseling and Psychotherapy*, marked developments could be found. In 1946 in his article entitled 'Significant aspects of client-centered therapy', Carl Rogers was still writing of 'non-directive' therapy and 'counselor techniques and procedures', and although he did acknowledge the influences of Freud, Rank, Taft and Allen, he also dismissed eclectic approaches as being 'not so fruitful'. He was able to state that, derived from practical clinical experience, there had been for him a movement *away from* guiding and directing and *towards* new ways of being (often seen as 'heretic' by other approaches to therapy) that seemed more helpful in terms of bringing about a meaningful therapeutic process. He identified three distinctive elements of what was beginning to be termed client-centred counselling, namely a *predictable process*, a *trust in the capacity of clients*, and *the therapist/client relationship*.

Predictable process

Carl Rogers stated that *if* a relationship founded on certain characteristics is initiated, *then* a predictable chain of events unfolds. At this time, he identified six elements (or 'conditions') necessary to bring about an experience within which the growth forces within clients are most likely to be tapped. These were that the counsellor:

1 holds a belief that individuals are responsible for themselves and is willing for people to keep self-responsibility
2 trusts in the growth forces within individuals, rather than in counsellor expertise and knowledge
3 creates a warm and permissive atmosphere within which clients are free to explore (or withhold) anything they wish to
4 sets limits only on behaviours, not on feelings or attitudes (deemed mostly relevant to working with children)
5 uses only procedures and techniques that convey deep understanding (such as 'sensitive reflection and clarification'), and does not express approval or disapproval
6 remains committed to working within the above five principles, in that the

counsellor does not question, probe, blame, interpret, advise, suggest, persuade or reassure.

Rogers maintained that whether the therapeutic process is relatively shallow or relatively deep, client-centred characteristics are fundamentally the same.

The capacity of the client

What made the therapeutic process predictable for Rogers was the discovery that:

> within the client reside constructive forces whose strength and uniformity have been either entirely unrecognized or grossly underestimated.
>
> (Rogers 1946: p. 417)

Carl had come to believe that clients, due to their tendencies to actualise, are *capable* of many things – such as beneficial emotional release at their own time and pace, effective self-exploration (even of denied feelings and attitudes), looking after their psychological selves, exploring the connections between self and non-self, and being strong and resourceful enough to come up with steps towards a positive journey through life. *If* the counsellor initiates a client-centred relationship, *then* all of these things become more likely. In stating that the more deeply the therapist trusts in the constructive forces within individuals the more deeply these tendencies are connected with, Rogers placed this emerging client-centred approach at an 'opposite pole' – both theoretically and practically – to the 'omnipotent counsellor with supernatural wisdom'. Rogers said that he now knew:

> that the client knows the areas of concern which he is ready to explore; that the client is the best judge as to the most desirable frequency of interviews; that the client can lead the way more efficiently than the therapist into deeper concerns; that the client will protect himself from panic by ceasing to explore an area which is becoming too painful; that the client can and will uncover all of the repressed elements which it is necessary to uncover in order to build a comfortable adjustment; that the client can achieve for himself far truer and more sensitive and accurate insights than can possibly be given to him; that the client is capable of translating these insights into constructive behavior which weigh his own needs and desires realistically against the demands of society; that the client knows when therapy is completed and he is ready to cope with life independently. Only one condition is necessary for all these forces to be released, and that is the proper psychological atmosphere between client and therapist.
>
> (Rogers 1946: pp. 418–19)

How different 'the client will protect himself from panic by ceasing to explore an area which is becoming too painful' feels to identifying *resistance* that must be overcome by the therapist, or *avoidance* that the analyst must circumvent in some way! The therapist can empathise, understand, accept, be with and, as a consequence, *move through* such phases *alongside* the client, rather than challenging, overcoming or circumventing. Another issue arising from this trust in the capacity of the client might be to question how 'the client knows when therapy is completed' fits with the introduction of *time-limited* therapy, which many believe to be driven by economic rather than therapeutic considerations. (Incidentally, figures from several sources indicate that where therapy is *not* time-limited, the average number of sessions per client is no more than six. This raises the question of why many service providers insist that client time must be managed, when philosophically, therapeutically and economically there would seem to be evidence that clients do indeed know best what is beneficial.) (e.g. Budman and Gurman 1988; Tolman 1990; Mellor-Clark *et al.* 2001.)

Client-centred therapy is so named because of the trust in and primary reliance upon the internal resources of the client, and Rogers believed that:

> There is no other aspect of client-centered therapy which comes under such vigorous attack. It seems to be genuinely disturbing to many professional people to entertain the thought that this client upon whom they have been exercising their professional skill actually knows more about his inner psychological self than they can possibly know, and that he possesses constructive strengths which make the constructive push by the therapist seem puny indeed by comparison. The willingness fully to accept this strength of the client, with all the re-orientation of therapeutic procedure which it implies, is one of the ways in which client-centered therapy differs most sharply from other therapeutic approaches.
>
> (Rogers 1946: p. 419)

Client-centred therapeutic relationships

Unlike therapies in which the counsellor uses skills, techniques and expertise upon clients, in client-centred work the fundamental starting point is the creation of an atmosphere within which clients may choose to grow. Carl identified some of the characteristics of such a relationship. For instance, clients would experience it as safe, warm, understanding and accepting. He also stated that 'the sense of communication' was a very important factor, in that not only could clients communicate anything they wished to, but also such communications would be understood rather than evaluated in any way. *The therapy session really does belong to the client.* Rogers quoted a Minister in counselling training as saying that one of the difficulties (trainee) therapists may face is when clients believe that the counsellor ought to be able to offer guidance – and the therapist values client-centred theory yet wonders whether it is enough, whether it goes far enough in actual practice. How can one leave a person struggling and helpless when one could help them by showing them the way out? The Minister posed some fundamental questions:

> Do you believe that all people truly have a creative potential in them? That each person is a unique individual and that he alone can work out his own individuality? Or do you really believe that some persons are of 'negative value' and others are weak and must be led and taught by 'wiser, stronger' people?

> In other methods you can shape tools, pick them up for use when you will. But when genuine acceptance and permissiveness are your tools it requires nothing less than the whole complete personality. And to grow oneself is the most demanding of all.
>
> (Rogers, 1946: p. 420)

Rogers wrote that the use of the term 'client-centred' arose through therapy being more effective the more the therapist strives to understand clients as clients experience themselves.

By 1946, Carl Rogers had realised that traces of 'subtle directiveness' were still to be found, and thus there was an increasing emphasis on the therapist discarding the need to diagnose (together with a personal need to display 'diagnostic shrewdness'), professional evaluations and prognoses, and the need to guide the client in order to be helpful. Rather, the client-centred therapist would strive to *provide understanding of the way the client seems to himself at this moment*, and the client would have the capacity to 'do the rest'. Rogers wrote:

> Client-centered counseling, if it is to be effective, cannot be a trick or a tool. It is not a subtle way of guiding the client while pretending to let him guide himself. To be *effective*, it must be genuine.
>
> (Rogers 1946: p. 420)

An authentically client-centred therapeutic relationship creates a 'psychological atmosphere which releases, frees, and utilises deep strengths in the client'.

Somewhere in between

Sigmund Koch invited Carl to contribute to his series of books entitled *Psychology: a study of a science*, and Carl had been wondering whether his developmental learning and growth might be drawn together into a consistent and understandable framework. We have already heard that he put a great deal of effort into this piece of work (*see* Prelude), and recalled:

> As one young psychologist with a background in mathematics said to me recently, 'It is so precise! I could restate it in mathematical terms.' I must confess this is close to my opinion.
>
> (Rogers and Evans 1981: pp. 135–6)

Yet Carl was puzzled and it *is* puzzling: his most rigorous piece of hard work being the most thoroughly ignored. Let us ignore it no longer!

Rogers gave us many important and fundamental definitions within his 1959 chapter, several of which follow. Given that the very term client-centred arose from the primary focus on the internal frame of reference of the person seeking help, let us begin there.

Internal frame of reference

> This is all of the realm of experience which is available to the awareness of the individual at a given moment. It includes the full range of sensations, perceptions, meanings, and memories which are

available to consciousness. The internal frame of reference is the subjective world of the individual. Only he knows it fully. It can never be known to another except through empathic inference, and then can never be perfectly known.

(Rogers 1959: p. 210)

The only way that I can *internally* validate my own experience is to focus further on my experiencing – to question, probe, examine, explore and reflect upon myself. If I attempt to check out my feelings with others, I observe myself as an object and thus am viewing myself from *external* reference points. As we shall see by and by, Rogers was to define the *process* of empathising as 'perception-checking', and the origins of this can be seen here:

> Knowledge which has any 'certainty', in the social sense, involves the use of empathic inference as a means of checking, but the direction of that empathy differs. When the experience of empathic understanding is used as a source of knowledge, one checks one's empathic inferences with the subject, thus verifying or disproving the inferences and hypotheses implicit in such empathy. It is this way of knowing which we have found so fruitful in therapy.
>
> (Rogers 1959: pp. 211–12)

External frame of reference

To perceive another person (or object) *without* empathising is to operate from an external frame of reference. Viewing objects in this way is common. Rarely, for instance, do we experience empathy for the chairs we sit upon, or the clothes we wear, or the pavements we walk along, or for the pen or word-processing equipment we use to write with! It could be said that none of these objects have any awareness of their own experiencing with which it would be possible to empathise. However, if *people* are viewed in the same way as objects (as, sadly, they so often seem to be, both from within and from outside the 'caring professions'), then human beings too become like inanimate objects.

An example comes to mind. A trainee counsellor on a client-centred course who was on placement with a bereavement service had been taught by that agency that there were five stages of grieving which clients needed to go through (and within a limited time frame, too). Counsellors were encouraged to identify the stage a client was in and attempt to move them on to the next stage, then the next, and so on. No attention at all was paid to fully receiving clients in the moment, and little attention was given to the inner world of client experiencing – little respect was shown for the capacity of clients to creatively discover their own constructive processes. Clients became objectified (in effect, a group of people had been pathologised) – they had to fit a model and both the therapist and the bereaved client needed to work in a way and at a pace dictated by that model. Furthermore, the model was somewhat white and Eurocentric, and if the bereaved client was not 'sorted' by having moved (or more accurately, by having been moved by the counsellor) through all five stages within the set time limit, their grieving was deemed to be 'abnormal' and subject to possible psychiatric referral.

Empathy

> The state of empathy, or being empathic, is to perceive the internal
> frame of reference of another with accuracy, and with the emotional
> components and meanings which pertain thereto, as if one were the
> other person, but without ever losing the 'as if' condition. Thus it
> means to sense the hurt or the pleasure of another as he senses it, and
> to perceive the causes thereof as he perceives them, but without ever
> losing the recognition that it is *as if* I were hurt or pleased, etc. If this 'as
> if' quality is lost, then the state is one of identification.
>
> (Rogers 1959: pp. 210–11)

A theory of therapy: if–then

Carl Rogers described the theory of client-centred therapy as being of the *if–then*
variety, even 'reverting' to theoretical logic:

$$B = (f)A \qquad C = (f)A \qquad B + C = (f)A \qquad C = (f)B$$

In the above formula, (f) represents *is a function of*, A denotes *conditions of the
therapeutic process*, B denotes *the process of therapy* and C denotes *outcomes in
personality and behaviour*. In other words, *if* (A) two persons are in contact, one
(the client) being incongruent and the other (the therapist) being congruent,
respectful and empathic, and the client perceives the therapist's unconditional
positive regard and empathic understanding at least to a minimal degree, *then* as a
consequence there will be (B), a therapeutic process. Also, *if* (A) *then* there will as
another consequence be predictable outcomes in terms of personal growth. Thus
both therapeutic process (B) and personal growth (C) are *functions of* the six
necessary and sufficient conditions. Likewise, predictable outcomes in terms
of personality change (C) are a consequence of (A), the necessary and sufficient
conditions. Rogers restated this by saying that the necessary and sufficient
conditions are independent variables, and client-centred therapeutic process
depends upon their existence. Thus (B) is a dependent variable. Once (B)
(therapeutic process) exists, then it becomes the independent variable, and (C)
(outcomes) are dependent variables. We can note, too, the idea that the greater
the degree of the existence of the necessary and sufficient conditions, the more
profound the process and outcomes are likely to be.

Necessary and sufficient

Carl Rogers believed that client-centred therapy differed markedly from conventional therapies, in that not only had *necessary* conditions been identified, but also
these conditions were deemed to be *sufficient*. He wrote that irrespective of the
particular characteristics of clients:

> It has been our experience to date that although the therapeutic
> relationship is used differently by different clients, it is not necessary
> or helpful to manipulate the relationship in specific ways for specific
> kinds of clients. To do this damages, it seems to us, the most helpful

and significant aspect of the experience, that it is a genuine relationship between two persons, each of whom is endeavoring, to the best of
his ability, to be himself in the interaction.

(Rogers 1959: pp. 213–14)

Having defined conditions that were both necessary and sufficient, Carl then
wondered *which* of the therapist conditions was the more important. He comes to
the conclusion that:

> For therapy to occur the wholeness of the therapist in the relationship
> is primary, but a part of the congruence of the therapist must be the
> experience of unconditional positive regard and the experience of
> empathic understanding.
>
> (Rogers 1959: p. 215)

This cannot be over-emphasised. It is simply not enough for the therapist to *be*
congruent. Client-centred congruence has little meaning or value unless unconditional positive regard and empathic understanding are fundamentally
embedded aspects that permeate the therapist's way of being, and that are
therefore authentically experienced by the therapist and may be perceived as
genuine by clients. However, to live by such profound attitudinal values towards
others in a sustained way might not be possible or even desirable (the therapist
has needs, wishes and rights, too). So Rogers also considered it important to note
that client-centred theory focuses upon conditions *within the therapeutic relationship,* pointing out that if it were to be necessary for the client-centred therapist to
be congruent at all times, there would be no client-centred therapists!

> Thus it is that imperfect human beings can be of therapeutic assistance
> to other imperfect human beings.
>
> (Rogers 1959: p. 215)

The actualising tendency

Carl Rogers also referred to the fundamental place in client-centred therapy of the
actualising tendency, which he defined as:

> the inherent tendency of the organism to develop all its capacities in
> ways which serve to maintain or enhance the organism.
>
> (Rogers 1959: p. 196)

Carl believed that certain therapeutic consequences of a belief in the actualising
tendency were inescapable, as:

> It means that psychotherapy is the releasing of an already existing
> capacity in a potentially competent individual, not the expert manip-
> ulation of a more or less passive personality. Philosophically it means
> that the individual has the capacity to guide, regulate and control
> himself, providing only that certain definable conditions exist.
>
> (Rogers 1959: p. 221)

The belief that human beings are, by their inner natures, constructive and
trustworthy was passionately held by Carl, who stated that:

> For me this is an inescapable conclusion from a quarter-century of experience in psychotherapy.
>
> (Rogers, 1957b: p. 299)

Rogers believed that there was no need to devise therapies based on control or socialisation, for when free from defensiveness, humans can be trusted to be positive, forward-moving, constructive, social beings who display deep needs for affiliation and communication with others. Humans have innate needs to like, love, respect and care for others beneath their sometimes more superficial hostile or aggressive behaviours. Indeed, such 'negative' actions are often the result of a squashing or thwarting of our fundamental natures. Carl wrote:

> I have little sympathy with the rather prevalent concept that man is basically irrational, and that his impulses, if not controlled, will lead to destruction of others and self. Man's behavior is exquisitely rational, moving with subtle and ordered complexity toward the goals his organism is endeavoring to achieve. The tragedy for most of us is that our defenses keep us from being aware of this rationality, so that consciously we are moving in one direction, while organismically we are moving in another.
>
> (Rogers 1957b: p. 300)

In other words, the internal barriers created by our incongruence serve to thwart our ability to be fully functioning individuals.

By 1967, the research of Carl Rogers and his colleagues (in this instance, Eugene Gendlin, Donald Kiesler and Charles Truax) was focused on such questions as 'What do we as therapists do that actually leads to constructive change in our clients or patients?'. It had already been ascertained that only a small fraction of the events occurring in counselling sessions actually had any really significant therapeutic impact, so what were these key factors? Likewise, it had also become clear that therapeutic relationships differ from therapist to therapist, *and* that an individual therapist will be different with different clients, *and* that an individual therapist will differ over time with the same client. Thus a therapist might adopt different language styles (from 'restricted' to 'elaborate') with different clients, and might move from gentle, tentative communications in early sessions with a client to more confident, understanding communications in later sessions with that same client. This would seem to give strong support to the client-centred belief that attitudes rather than behaviours are most relevant to the process of therapy.

Rogers pointed out that many writers from many orientations (psychoanalysts Ferenczi, Alexander, Schafer, Halpern and Lesser, and eclectic writers Strunk, Raush and Bordin, Strupp, Hobbs, Fox and Gordin) as well as client-centred authors (Dymond, Jourard, Truax, and Rogers himself) had stressed the importance of:

> the therapist's ability to understand sensitively and accurately the inner experiences of the client or patient, . . . the maturity of the therapist and his integration or genuineness within the relationship . . . [and] warmth and his acceptance of the individual with whom [the

therapist] is working . . . Cutting across parochial viewpoints, they can be considered as elements common to a wide variety of therapies.

(Rogers 1967: p. 98)

Thus we were again reminded of what became known as the three 'core' or therapist conditions for client-centred therapy. Rogers emphasised that all three of these common elements were 'logically intertwined'. For instance, while empathic understanding is essential, it is a prior requirement that acceptance and prizing be present if a therapist is to be 'deeply sensitive to the moment-to-moment "being" of another person'. While unconditional positive regard is necessary for empathy, neither have much meaning unless they are authentic.

Congruence

Rogers pointed out that we are unlikely to reveal our inner selves to people who 'put up a front' or play a role (e.g. a professional façade) or feign understanding – in other words, we are not likely to go too far or too deep with incongruent (inauthentic or phony) people. We are more likely to share with therapists who are *being*, not *denying* (or distorting) who they are, and where a striving to be respectful and empathic is deeply embedded within that way of being. In an attempt to circumvent misunderstanding, Carl also clarified some of the things that being congruent does *not* mean. For instance, it does not mean that therapists overtly express all of their feelings (thereby over-burdening clients), nor does it mean an impulsive blurting out of feelings without thought, nor does it mean total therapist self-disclosure.

Congruence *does* mean that the therapist does not *deny* any experienced feelings, and that there is a willingness to *transparently be* any persistent feelings that arise within the relationship, and to *communicate* them within the relationship *if appropriate*. When might it be appropriate to share such feelings? For Carl, this would seem to be either if the feeling persists over time or if the feeling gets in the way of deeply hearing a client. When it *is* appropriate to share such feelings, Rogers stated that it was important for the therapist to *own* them (rather than 'project' them on to the client). The client-centred therapist being in touch with inner experiencing is ongoing, and this can be communicated, too. Thus the discomfort in or anxiety about sharing the feeling can accompany the feeling itself. This, stated Rogers, enables the relationship to grow and become more real.

Thus if a therapist feels boredom and communicates this to a client (owning the feeling and their apprehension about sharing the feeling), it emerges that the therapist experiences distance from the client and would like to connect more deeply. The boredom – a barrier – dissipates and a new sensitivity emerges. It may be that the therapist becomes more able to deeply hear the client again – even to hear the client's shock or hurt at what has been said. Both client and therapist will be more genuine as a consequence of the therapist daring to be real. Carl Rogers said that there had been a gradual shift between 1950 and the mid to late 1960s, and that client-centred counsellors had come to feel increasingly free about being 'whole persons' in the therapeutic encounter. Carl said that his 'trial ground' for being more fully himself (for reasons that he did not fully understand) was working with groups, within which:

I express anger, and affection, and annoyance and all kinds of things, as well as being very responsive to hurt. Hurt arouses in me feelings of really wanting to be empathic so that a lot of the therapeutic attitudes that I've stressed, I think, are very real parts of me, and of many therapists, and so they need expression as well, but other feelings, too, have equal validity.

(Rogers 1969, in Frick 1989: p. 102)

It may be that therapists struggle more with the communication of feelings that are experienced, anticipated or heard as being *negative*. Ideally, it might possibly be said that the therapist would only experience positive attitudes – yet if this is not the case, Rogers believed that it is harmful to clients if such feelings are hidden. He considered that every therapist has negative attitudes from time to time, but that it is preferable for them to be expressed, and for the counsellor to be real, not false.

In my relationships with persons I have found that it does not help, in the long run, to act as though I were something that I am not. It does not help to act calm and pleasant when actually I am angry and critical. It does not help to act as though I know the answers when I do not. It does not help to act as though I were a loving person if actually, at the moment, I am hostile. It does not help for me to act as though I were full of assurance, if actually I am frightened and unsure.

(Rogers 1961: p. 16)

Why might it be appropriate or reasonable for therapists to share persistent feelings that arise within the therapeutic relationship with their clients? According to Carl Rogers, it is because:

It is not an easy thing for the client, or for any human being, to trust his most deeply shrouded feelings to another person. It is even more difficult for a disturbed person to share his deepest and most troubling feelings with a therapist. The genuineness, or congruence, of the therapist is one of the elements in the relationship which makes this risk of sharing easier and less fraught with dangers.

(Rogers 1967: p. 102)

Carl Rogers gave some possible indicators of therapist *incongruence*. They included defensiveness (which might be apparent through inconsistencies between therapist words and paraverbal or non-verbal communicating), or making 'textbook responses' that are intended to sound good rather than being expressions of authentic, respectful empathy. Rogers identified voice qualities and manner of expression as the most usual indicators of congruence, saying that it was fortunate that we are all pretty adept at distinguishing between the authentic and the phony. Carl did become increasingly concerned about the frequent misunderstanding of the notion of therapist self-expression within the concept of congruence, writing that:

it does not mean that the therapist burdens his client with overt expression of all his feelings. Nor does it mean that the therapist discloses his total self to his client. It does mean, however, that the therapist denies to himself none of the feelings he is experiencing and that he is willing to experience transparently any *persistent* feelings that exist in the relationship and to let these be known to his client. It means avoiding the temptation to present a façade or hide behind a mask of professionalism, or to assume a confessional–professional attitude.

(Rogers 1989: pp. 11–13)

Unconditional positive regard

The attitude of high regard held by the client-centred counsellor for the dignity and worth of individuals is a fundamental differentiation between client-centred therapy and a great many other approaches. This had come to mean that, *without reservation*, the therapist *experienced and communicated* a non-judgemental, acceptant warmth, a deep and genuine caring, and a non-evaluative 'pure' ('uncontaminated') prizing of client feelings, thoughts or behaviours. This deep respect for clients included a trust in both their capacity and their right to self-direction (underpinned by a trust in the actualising tendency).

Rogers stated that, as therapists, we might even find painful and negative client expressions easier to accept than good or positive ones, yet *unconditional* positive regard means the acceptance of *all* expressions – no 'ifs' or 'buts' – it is a *non-possessive caring for the client as a separate person*. Yet so often, it seems, we hear phrases like 'I accept the person but not their behaviour', though as Carl said, 'it is doubtful if this is an adequate or true comment', in that although a client behaviour may feel 'bad' or socially unacceptable to a therapist, there is a kind of 'there but for the grace of god' element in acceptance: the behaviour is accepted 'as a *natural consequence* of the circumstances, experiences, and feelings of this client'. By providing a non-threatening climate within which clients are able to choose to explore their inner selves (rather than approving or disapproving), the therapist becomes a companion searching with the client for *client* meanings and values.

Carl Rogers believed that many people who are striving to become client-centred therapists do so because:

> [their] philosophical orientation has tended to move in the direction of greater respect for the individual.
>
> (Rogers 1951: p. 21)

Becoming a client-centred therapist offers an opportunity to put this philosophical belief into practice. Such a trainee counsellor:

> soon learns that the development of the way of looking upon people which underlies this therapy is a continuing process, closely related to the therapist's own struggle for personal growth and integration. He can be only as 'nondirective' as he has achieved respect for others in his own personality organization.
>
> (Rogers 1951: p. 21)

Thus a link emerges between congruence and unconditional positive regard, for as Carl stated time and time again, respect for clients needs to be a deeply integrated, fundamental and integral aspect of the therapist's personality. On the one hand, experiencing deep respect for another can be deeply enriching and energising for the therapist. On the other hand, it can be a strenuous and problematic struggle:

> *I have found it highly rewarding when I can accept another person.* I have found that truly to accept another person and his feelings is by no means an easy thing, any more than is understanding. Can I really permit another person to feel hostile toward me? Can I accept his anger as a real and legitimate part of himself? Can I accept him when he views life and its problems in a way quite different from mine? Can I accept him when he feels very positively toward me, admiring me and wanting to model himself after me? All this is involved in acceptance, and it does not come easy.
>
> (Rogers 1961: pp. 20–21)

The more acceptance the therapist experiences and offers, the more a useful helping relationship exists:

> By acceptance I mean a warm regard for him as a person of uncondi-tional self-worth – of value no matter what his condition, his behavior, or his feelings. It means a respect and liking for him as a separate person, a willingness for him to possess his own feelings in his own way. It means an acceptance of and regard for his attitudes of the moment, no matter how negative or positive, no matter how much they may contradict other attitudes he has held in the past. This acceptance of each fluctuating aspect of this other person makes it for him a relationship of warmth and safety, and the safety of being liked and prized as a person seems a highly important element in a helping relationship.
>
> (Rogers 1961: p. 34)

Accurate empathic understanding

Empathic understanding also needs to be deeply embedded within the personality of the counsellor:

> In client-centered therapy the client finds in the counselor a genuine alter ego in an operational and technical sense – a self which has temporarily divested itself (so far as possible) of its own selfhood, except for the one quality of endeavoring to understand.
>
> (Rogers 1951: p. 40)

Carl Rogers offered us a challenge, and through trying this we could test the degree of our empathic understanding:

> The next time you get into an argument with your wife, or your friend, or with a small group of friends, just stop the discussion for a moment and for an experiment, institute this rule. 'Each person can speak up for himself only *after* he has first restated the ideas and feelings of the previous speaker accurately, and to that speaker's satisfaction.' You see

what this would mean. It would simply mean that before presenting your own point of view, it would be necessary for you to really achieve the other speaker's frame of reference – to understand his thoughts and feelings so well that you could summarize them for him. Sounds simple, doesn't it? But if you try it you will discover it is one of the most difficult things you have ever tried to do.

(Rogers 1961: p. 332)

Once therapist congruence and unconditional positive regard *are* present:

The ability of the therapist accurately and sensitively to understand experiences and feelings *and their meaning to the client* during the moment-to-moment encounter of psychotherapy constitutes what can perhaps be described as the 'work' of the therapist

(Rogers 1967: p. 104)

Rogers identified two major aspects of empathic understanding, namely *immediacy* and *communication*. Over the years it seems as though there have been many interpretations of the term 'immediacy', including the therapist spontaneously blurting out every passing feeling (which Carl so much disliked). What Carl Rogers meant by this term was that *immediacy in experiencing empathy* was a necessity. After all, it is of little use if the therapist only achieves insight or feels completely at home in the universe of the client some time after the counselling session has ended (for example, in the car on the way home!). The capacity to sensitively communicate client inner meanings back to the client in such a way that they *belong* to the client – and in a language *attuned* to the client – was the other crucial factor for effective client-centred therapy. Such communicating serves to clarify and expand client awareness of feelings or experiences, and includes the 'sensitive play of voice qualities which reflect the seriousness, the intentness, and the depth of feeling' as well as the actual words used.

Rogers again differentiated between *internal* and *external* frames of reference. At that time, the most common form of understanding in therapies other than client-centred was an external, even impersonal, evaluative diagnostic formulation that implied 'I know what is wrong with you' (an understanding from the outside looking in), as compared with 'an accurate and sensitive grasp of events and experiences and their *personal meaning to the client*' (in other words, an understanding from within the world of client feelings and meanings). Carl offered us questions that he had found useful when exploring the degree to which he could permit himself to experience empathy. They included the following:

Can I let myself enter fully into the world of his feelings and personal meanings and see these as he does? Can I step into his private world so completely that I lose all desire to evaluate or judge it? Can I enter it so sensitively that I can move about in it freely, without trampling on meanings which are precious to him? Can I sense it so accurately that I can catch not only the meanings of his experience which are obvious to him, but those meanings which are only implicit, which he sees only dimly or as confusion? Can I extend this understanding without limit?

(Rogers 1961: pp. 53–4)

Rogers also pointed out that the communication of *striving* to understand can in itself be therapeutic – if nothing else, it both lets clients know that they are *worth* the effort, and encourages them to communicate further. However, a consistent inability to do more than strive might not be so helpful. Indeed, if the therapist does not *achieve* accurate empathic understanding over a significant period, a consequence may be that the client feels ever more helpless and despairing.

Carl also gave some pointers to factors characteristic of low, intermediate, high and very high levels of empathy. At the *extremely negative* end of the scale, the therapist shows no comprehension at all of the feelings and meanings that the client is trying to communicate, and *fairly negative* elements included the therapist being perceived as hostile, superior, and even disgusted. Clues to *low levels* of empathy included the therapist going off at a tangent, communicating only the client's most obvious feelings, misinterpreting, being intellectually preoccupied, attending to content rather than what the client is experiencing in each moment, evaluating, giving advice, using inappropriate language or timing, or reflecting upon therapist experiencing rather than the client's experiencing.

Intermediate levels of empathy are indicated by the therapist accurately sensing and communicating the client's most obvious feelings, yet only occasionally sensing and communicating less apparent ones. In so doing, the counsellor 'may anticipate feelings that are not current or may misinterpret the present feelings'.

High levels of empathy are indicated by the therapist communicating deeper yet slightly inaccurate awareness of feelings and experiences – 'pointing' to more hidden feelings yet 'unable to grasp their meaning':

> At a *very high level of empathic understanding* [my italics] the therapist's responses move, with sensitivity and accuracy, into feelings and experiences that are only hinted at by the client. At this level, underlying feelings or experiences are not only pointed to, but they are specifically identified so that the content that comes to light may be new but it is not alien. At this high level the therapist is sensitive to his own tentative errors and quickly alters or changes his responses in midstream, indicating a clear but fluid responsiveness to what is being sought after in the patient's own explorations. The therapist's words reflect a togetherness with the patient and a tentative trial-and-error exploration, while his voice tone reflects the seriousness and depth of his empathic grasp.
>
> (Rogers 1967: p. 106)

Rogers was interested in the findings of two research programmes undertaken by Fiedler, who found that therapists who were able to totally engage with client communications were most characteristic of a good therapeutic relationship, followed by accurate therapist comments, co-operative therapists, power equality, good therapist understanding, consistent striving to understand, accurate tracking of the client, and a sharing tone of voice (Rogers 1951: pp. 53–4). The theme of levels of empathy is explored more fully in Chapter 4.

Empathic understanding enriches both therapist and client, for as Rogers wrote:

> When I can permit myself to understand . . . it is mutually rewarding. And with clients in therapy, I am often impressed with the fact that even a minimal amount of empathic understanding – a bumbling and faulty attempt to catch the confused complexity of the client's mean-ing – is helpful, though there is no doubt that it is most helpful when I can see and formulate clearly the meanings in his experiencing which for him have been unclear and tangled.
>
> (Rogers 1961: p. 54)

Towards the end

Carl Rogers stated the obvious – that all approaches to counselling and psy-chotherapy have a focus on clients. However, he also stated that in client-centred therapy there is a seldom explicated technical connotation, in that while in most approaches achieving understanding of clients is seen as a step towards eliciting a case history for future reference and analysis, or behaviour modification or re-education or whatever (the 'real work' of such therapists):

> Instead, the client-centered therapist aims to remain with this phe-nomenal universe throughout the entire course of therapy and holds that stepping outside it – to offer external interpretations, to give advice, to suggest, to judge – only retards therapeutic gain.
>
> (Rogers 1989: p. 21)

In 1980, Carl wrote that he was so shocked and appalled at the way empathy had become known as a set of techniques (like 'reflecting' or 'mirroring'), and had become such an insulting caricature of what was in fact 'one of the most delicate and powerful ways we have of using ourselves', that for many years he had written or said little on the subject. Then he wrote *In Retrospect: Forty-Six Years* because he was:

> getting tired of the misunderstanding of the concept of empathy, of superficial notions such as saying back to the person what they said and things like that.
>
> (Rogers and Russell 2002: p. 211)

In reminiscing, Carl remembered how in his earlier days he had learned that 'simply listening' to a client was helpful:

> Yet listening, of this very special kind, is one of the most potent forces for change that I know.
>
> (Rogers 1980: p. 116)

However, the phrase 'simply listening' might be a little misleading:

> I think that one of the elements most likely to be misunderstood is the intensity of empathic listening. People feel, you know, that listening is a sort of passive experience. I feel that's one thing that's badly

> misunderstood . . . One of the complexities of the person-centered approach is that in many ways it is a very disciplined approach . . . And there's a discipline involved in helping to make that shift [into the client's world]; there's a discipline involved in being deeply empathic. It means you really do shut things out, and you are focused. Because the essence of it is simple, people forget that there is also disciplined learning and disciplined action in the interaction.
>
> (Rogers and Russell 2002: p. 284)

Then, when Rogers moved to Teachers College, Columbia University, he learned (from Elizabeth Davies or Leta Hollingworth – he quoted Elizabeth in Rogers and Raskin (1989) and Leta in Rogers (1985) – both Rankian social workers) that listening for feelings and emotions was effective, and that these feelings could be 'reflected back' to the client. Although he expressed gratitude for this as it improved his work at that time, he also wrote of:

> 'Reflect' becoming in time a word that made me cringe.
>
> (Rogers 1980: p. 138)

Rogers then moved to Ohio State University, and the recording of counselling sessions began. Although he believed throughout his life that the recording and analysis of interviews is one of the best routes to self-improvement as a therapist, and although a great deal of client-centred theory was derived from such 'microscopic' studies, there were deeply regrettable consequences, especially in terms of a focus on skills and techniques, as compared with 'a *way of being* that is rarely seen in full bloom in a relationship'.

So for many years Rogers spoke and wrote only of empathic attitude rather than of how empathic attitudes might be communicated, choosing to focus instead on congruence and unconditional positive regard because, he said, although they too were 'often misunderstood . . . at least they were not caricatured'. Only in 1980 did he return to commenting on how an empathic attitude might be *implemented*. He stated that in part this was due to his view that an increasingly technological society was breeding approaches to therapy (citing gestalt, psychodrama, primal therapy, bioenergetics, rational–emotive therapy and transactional analysis as examples) in which the *therapist* was very much the expert and which involved clients being actively manipulated, whereas he believed empathy to be 'possibly the most potent factor in bringing about change and learning', and that an empathic way of being empowered rather than disempowered clients.

Experiencing

Carl Rogers referred to Eugene Gendlin, who formulated the view that at all times human beings can refer to their ongoing inner experiencing. The client-centred therapist accurately gathers this 'felt meaning', and the perceiving of this by clients helps them to focus further on such meanings. Thus clients can access this 'ongoing psycho-physiological flow within' and use it as an inner referent (hence 'internal frame of reference'). Carl said that this psychophysiological flow is very real:

It's the kind of process that enables the therapist to be really in touch with the correct words that are going on in the client's mind . . . One word will not fit; another one that seems quite similar may absolutely fit. It's as though there's some physiological click, and you can see it in the client's face and manner of expression: 'No, that's not quite it; yes, that's it'. Their response indicates whether it is a click or not.

(Rogers and Russell 2002: p. 254)

Imagine, if you will, the therapist venturing an empathic communication: 'You seem angry . . .'. The client pauses a moment, and says, 'Kind of . . . Maybe more *frustrated* than angry . . .'. What is the client *doing* during the pause? When *I* pause in this way, I am taking a few moments to sort of 'stop' myself, or 'freeze-frame' – and I kind of 'look inside myself' to see what is 'really' going on. Take a moment now – do it yourself and *see*.

> Thus the client-centered therapist aims to concentrate on the *immediate phenomenal world* of the client. For he believes that it is in confusions or contradictions within this world that the client's difficulties lie. This exclusive focus in therapy on the present phenomenal experience of the client is the meaning of the term 'client-centered'.
>
> (Rogers 1989: p. 22)

However, there is a difference of opinion among client-centred practitioners with regard to quite how this focus on the client's phenomenal world is implemented:

> Some aim to convey an understanding of just what the client wishes to communicate. For Rogers, it has felt right not only to clarify meanings of which the client is aware, but also those just below the level of awareness.
>
> (Rogers and Raskin 1989: p. 171)

Also:

> This is not to say, however, that the client-centered therapist responds only to the obvious in the phenomenal world of his client. If that were so, it is doubtful that any movement would ensue in therapy. Indeed, there would be no therapy. Instead, the client-centered therapist aims to dip from the pool of implicit meanings just at the edge of the client's awareness.
>
> (Rogers 1989: p. 21)

From such statements we can glean something of different levels of empathy within a therapeutic process. When speaking of the therapist being a companion to clients, Carl said:

> I think that the therapist's function is that of being a companion to the client in the client's search for the innermost aspects of self and experience. It is much easier to face a denied experience if someone is right with you.
>
> (Rogers and Russell 2002: pp. 281–2)

It is far better to journey with a *companion* than to travel alone . . .

In striving to 'track' a client, the therapist is sometimes a little way behind yet striving to be alongside, sometimes there is an equal reciprocity, and sometimes the therapist is aware of feelings and meanings only vaguely experienced or perceived by the client. We saw that being too far behind (being unempathic) is not at all helpful – being too far ahead can be hurtful, too. Carl Rogers was mindful of the work of radical psychoanalyst Heinz Kohut, and said:

> Similarly, way back in my early years of training young counselors, some of the most sensitive of them were so empathic that they understood material the client was not yet aware of, was quite frightened of. And when it was verbalized, the client vanished. We began to call them 'blitz therapists'. They had the makings of very good counselors, but they had to learn that you don't verbalize an understanding that is deeper than the client needs, or wants, or can deal with consciously.
>
> (Rogers and Teich 1992: p. 56)

From state to process

One development that was clear by 1980 was that Rogers had changed from writing about empathy as a *state of being* to defining empathy as a *way of being*, a *process*:

> An empathic way of being with another person has several facets. It means entering the private perceptual world of the other and becoming thoroughly at home in it. It involves being sensitive, moment by moment, to the changing felt meanings which flow in this other person, to the fear or rage or tenderness or confusion or whatever he or she is experiencing. It means temporarily living in the other's life, moving about in it delicately without making judgments; it means sensing meanings of which he or she is scarcely aware, but not trying to uncover totally unconscious feelings, since this would be too threatening. It includes communicating your sensings of the person's world as you look with fresh and unfrightened eyes at elements of which he or she is fearful. It means frequently checking with the person as to the accuracy of your sensings, and being guided by the responses you receive. You are a confident companion to the person in his or her inner world. By pointing to the possible meanings in the flow of another person's experiencing, you help the other to focus on this useful type of referent, to experience the meanings more fully, and to move forward in the experiencing.
>
> (Rogers 1980: p. 142)

Carl Rogers added:

> One thing that seems very true to me is that there is no such thing as a perception without a meaning. That is, the human organism immediately attaches a meaning to whatever is perceived . . . The world of reality for the individual is his own field of perception, with the meanings he has attached to those various aspects . . . None of us

knows for sure what constitutes objective reality and we live our whole lives in the reality as perceived.

(Rogers and Evans 1981: pp. 9–10)

Here then, yet again, we see a focus on both feelings *and meanings* as integral aspects of empathic understanding. We see, too, a more dynamic *process* of an *ongoing perception checking* of our empathic understanding than would be the case, say, with simply paraphrasing, or summarising, or asking 'open' questions, or reflecting (feelings or otherwise) in response to what a client has just said. Indeed, it might be helpful if trainee client-centred therapists were to eliminate the word 'response' from their therapeutic vocabulary – it could well be more fruitful to think in terms of striving to respectfully *communicate* empathic understanding than *respond* to what has just been said. It might be, too, that focusing on each individual counsellor 'response' carries with it the risk of empathy being seen as a *state* (any individual therapist communication being rated on a scale from empathic to non-empathic – a kind of 'in that moment it either is or is not empathic' approach), thereby losing sight of the flow, the *process,* the essence of an empathic *way of being* and a therapeutic, reciprocal relationship.

If would-be therapists simply learn to reflect, paraphrase, summarise and the like, there is a tragic loss of both unique individuality and potential. Research concludes that there is a great variety of counsellor communications, influenced by both the life history of a counsellor and their personal style. Individual therapists must *choose* each communication that they utter:

> Each therapist has his favorite themes, specific sensitivities, and degrees of high attunement. With each special attunement, there are characteristic areas of low emphasis in which each therapist is fairly opaque, insensitive, and even neglectful.
>
> (Barton 1974: p. 201)

Perhaps a couple of personal examples might be helpful at this point. As a humanist I do not believe in any God or gods, and I became aware that I was less sensitive and open to religious beliefs than I would ideally like to be; my experiences of the church and other religious establishments had also generated bias and prejudice. I have therefore had to work on my acceptance in these areas. On the other hand, being a male who once experienced a sexual assault (when I was 12 years old) has, I believe, served to sensitise me to clients who have been violated (although I have to be constantly vigilant in differentiating between empathy and identification). A third example might be worthy of mention. Often in training students decide to explore empathic communications (*not* reflecting or paraphrasing) in a group setting, and several different communications emerge in response to one client disclosure. Yet examine these varied communications, and many of them will be positively therapeutic – celebrate diversity!

To clarify yet further the range of empathic expressions available to individual therapists, we can turn to Peggy Natiello, who took a close look at a 30-minute session that a client called Mary had with Carl Rogers:

> Even in the half-hour relationship presented here, there is a subtle change and expansion of Rogers' style of response. Most of his responses are geared toward empathic understanding, but there is a

good deal of variety in the form they take. He asks direct questions to further his understanding; repeats what he thinks he is hearing, sometimes literally, sometimes metaphorically; links ideas from earlier in the session to later disclosures; completes the client's sentences; helps her find the right words; speaks in the first person as though he were her; and even jokes a little.

(Farber *et al.* 1996: p. 126)

Some trainees and practitioners struggle with the notion of therapists making choices each time they communicate to clients, for might this not imply that client-centred therapy is not so 'non-directive' as they had thought it to be? Maria Villa-Boas Bowen tackled Rogers on this very issue. He replied (in a personal communication, dated 16 January 1983):

When I try to respond to the feeling that is most important to the client, my choice of what is most important is certainly influenced by my own personality, past history, and so forth. I agree that that is most assuredly true and I don't think I have ever said [otherwise]. . . . If it is openly recognized that such responses are partly shaped by the therapist's *perception* and that this perception is shaped both by the client's expression and by the therapist's personality, we may be able to avoid imitative 'modeling'.

(Farber *et al.* 1996: pp. 90–91)

As we explore the various aspects involved in empathic understanding, we see once again the importance of the therapist being sensitive, non-judging and unafraid, for:

To be with another in this way means that for the time being, you lay aside your own views and values in order to enter another's world without prejudice. In some sense it means that you lay aside your self; this can only be done by persons who are secure enough in themselves that they know they will not get lost in what may turn out to be the strange or bizarre world of the other, and that they can comfortably return to their own world when they wish . . . being empathic is a complex, demanding, and strong – yet also a subtle and gentle – way of being.

(Rogers 1980: p. 143)

Here we might again make links with both *congruence* and *unconditional positive regard*, for only if this intense and respectful focus on the inner world of the client is a consequence of deeply held and integrated beliefs can it be deemed to be authentic – that is, congruent. I need to be *genuinely* interested in the world of feelings and meanings of the other, not simply playing a role or somehow pretending to be absorbed by the other. This suggests most strongly that if I am to become a client-centred therapist, then developing my own personal growth and awareness far outweighs the learning and implementation of 'non-directive' skills and techniques.

Gay (Swenson) Barfield quotes some of Rogers' 1980 definition when exploring empathy with him in a filmed exchange of views in 1985, in which Carl acknowledged the benefits of empathy in a variety of settings, such as the classroom, intimate relationships (such as marriage and parent/child relation-ships), hostile groups and international relations. Carl said:

> I know that many tensions exist because of failures in communication, and each group has arrived at the pattern of feeling: 'I'm right and you're wrong. I'm good and you're bad'. And the trouble is that the other group feels exactly the same way: 'I'm right and you're wrong. I'm good and you're bad'. This destroys communication; it is also a good example of an absolute lack of empathy.
>
> (Rogers and Teich 1992: p. 58)

However, Carl went on to mention his unhappiness at the misuse and abuse of empathy that has taken place, quoting counselling training programmes as an example of this – courses wherein 'wooden, mechanical' techniques of 'reflecting feelings' and paraphrasing are taught and learned, and there is a lack of sensitivity and affect. Indeed, Rogers recalled one trainer saying to him after a demonstra-tion session that only three or four of Carl's empathic 'responses' would have been acceptable on his course! Of empathy as a technique or skill, Rogers said:

> I regard that as not only a distortion but really a gross misunderstand-ing of the whole concept, that often turns out people who are not helpful at all as counselors.
>
> (Rogers and Barfield 1985)

Empathy, said Rogers, involves the whole person of the therapist intensely yet delicately (because of the possibility of hurt) focusing on the inner world of the client – so much so that an empathic way of being at its most intense was 'a slightly altered state of consciousness' in which the therapist is being a companion to clients as they explore, sometimes fearfully, their inner selves in search of new personal meanings and feelings. The inner world of another person is clearly 'not a place to move around like a bull in a china shop', and the therapist needs to be a *confident* companion in order not to be shocked or judging. Stating that truly being understood and sensing that you are *worth* understanding is a 'very precious feeling to have', Carl recalled a demonstration session with a therapist from a different approach, who said afterwards 'You know, I've heard all the jokes about client-centred therapy, but it feels *so good* to be *heard*'.

If we are not mechanically reflecting or paraphrasing or whatever, what are we doing when we empathise? Rogers described the process of empathy as checking one's perceptions *of* the client *with* the client, using different forms of speech and styles as appropriate. Indeed, Rogers often found himself speaking *for* the client as if he were in the client's inner world, stating that clients would soon let him know if he was inaccurate.

Intuition

It could be said that just as Carl Rogers implicitly trusted the innate resources and potential of clients, so he grew to trust his own capacities, too:

> As a therapist, I find that when I am closest to my inner, intuitive self, when I am somehow in touch with the unknown in me, when perhaps

> I am in a slightly altered state of consciousness in the relationship, then whatever I do seems to be full of healing.
>
> (Rogers *et al.* 1986: p. 130)

It is regrettable (in my view at least, although I know that I am not alone) that there are some who have argued that Rogers intended intuition to become an additional therapist condition, whereas he himself clearly placed his intuitive experiencing within the realm of empathic understanding. It is even more regrettable (again in my view, and again I am not alone) that some people have abused segments like 'the unknown in me' and 'slightly altered state of consciousness' in their attempts to argue that Carl intended to add spirituality as an additional therapist condition. As we shall see – hogwash!

Reciprocity

Carl and Gay also spoke of the *reciprocity* of empathy, saying that although in other relationships the experiencing and offering of empathy could be somewhat one-sided (and therefore unhealthy), in therapy, although it is the therapist who mostly offers empathy, the empathic process is not *entirely* one-directional. In essence, this means that the therapist relies on clients to empathise with and understand his or her empathic understanding of them – there is a reciprocal process. Thus 'two persons being in contact' and 'the client receives, at least to a minimal degree, the unconditional positive regard and empathic understanding of the therapist' (the first and sixth necessary and sufficient conditions) can be linked with the notion of reciprocity in empathic process. Another illustration of 'reciprocal empathy' is when the therapist chooses to express an apparently non-therapeutic or 'negative' feeling that has persisted in the counselling relationship, such as anger or boredom. Carl stated that in such moments the therapist relies on the empathy and understanding of the client to get through such phases.

Gender

Although it is difficult to find many references to gender issues in the writings of Carl Rogers, it might be of interest to note that in this interview with Gay Barfield, Rogers did comment on a trend, namely males becoming more acquainted with and accustomed to their 'softer' or more 'feminine' side, rather than simply being dominating and 'macho' men. It may be that this greater willingness of men to strive to be empathic and understanding is linked with a move away from more directive approaches to psychotherapy.

It is abundantly clear when watching the video *Empathy: an Exploration* that in his later years Rogers believed passionately that empathy was a compassionate, delicate and sensitive way to *be with* people, not some technique or skill to *use on* them.

Summary

What have we learned of empathic understanding by trawling through its origins and developments? Here are six headings:

1 Context
2 Clients are active, not passive
3 Being a person
4 Does not, is not
5 Empathic understanding is . . .
6 Predictable process and consequences.

Context

Empathic understanding occurs within the context of other necessary and sufficient conditions, namely being in meaningful contact with another person (the client), the other person being relatively incongruent, the therapist being congruent and experiencing unconditional positive regard and empathic understanding, and the client perceiving the unconditional positive regard and empathic understanding of the therapist. These conditions are both necessary and sufficient – client-centred therapy is not eclectic. Although it is true that therapeutic relationships can include broader applications of client-centred therapy, known as the person-centred approach, it is also a fact that Carl Rogers went so far as to state that the use of different techniques for different people in one-to-one therapy:

> goes a long way towards destroying the possibility of a growthful experience for clients.
>
> (Rogers and Sanford 1985)

Clients are active, not passive

At the heart of client-centred theory lies the *actualising tendency*, a belief that individuals have their own *inner* resources (which have traditionally been underestimated or even ignored). Clients are capable of setting their own time and pace in therapy (for beneficial emotional disclosure, for instance) and of self-exploring at self-controlled depth. Clients may be self-protecting (withdrawing when appropriate, as compared with resisting or avoiding) and, given the right conditions, are strong, resourceful, positive and constructive. Clients are capable of achieving insight, which in turn may lead to behavioural choices. Clients also know best when to end therapy. People have access to their experiencing and their inner psychophysiological flow, and thus have a capacity for organismic valuing. The *client* does the probing, examining, exploring and reflecting. The constructive capacity of clients is immense, and the efforts of the therapist are puny by comparison. The client-centred therapist goes to work *with* a client – not *on* one!

Being a person

The prime requisite for becoming a client-centred therapist is being a person – an imperfect, whole person is good enough. This person strives in a disciplined way to be delicately sensitive, true, honest, trustworthy, compassionate, secure, transparent, real, non-defensive, non-possessive, non-threatening, self-aware (of inner warps, biases and prejudices), aware of others and their social/cultural contexts, genuinely receptive and interested, caring, deeply understanding, warm and permissive, and engages only in appropriate self-disclosure. Unconditional positive regard (characterised by a 'there but for the grace of some deity go I' attitude) and empathic understanding *must* be integrated and owned parts of the congruence of the therapist, as must a respect for the sovereignty and autonomy of individuals and their potential capacities and resources.

Does not, is not

Such a person finds it impossible to moralise, be prejudicial, judge, be horrified, blame, interpret, probe, question (open or otherwise), advise, suggest, paraphrase, summarise, persuade, reassure, diagnose, evaluate, deliver prognoses, guide, manipulate, go off at a tangent, reflect on therapist (their own) experiencing, use inappropriate language, mirror, reflect, become lost or over-immersed in the other's inner world, project a professional façade or front, pretend or be otherwise phony, direct, criticise, approve or disapprove, praise, lose the essence of the I–thou relationship by focusing on a frozen state of empathy (individual 'responses', for example), be the expert or blurt out every passing feeling.

Technological society has tended to produce experts who use skills on people (going to work *on* clients, not *with* them). As a result, a regrettable caricature of empathic understanding arose. However, in client-centred therapy empathy is not at all to do with skills, techniques, tools, tricks, expertise or wooden, mechanical, textbook counsellor responses.

Tricks? The therapist *using tricks on people* conjures up the image of the conjurer. *Con* suggests manipulative, and a *juror* decides, or is judgemental. Why, expertly and professionally, pull this *technique* out of the hat, or that *skill* from up your sleeve, or suddenly wave your wand to make that *tool* appear as if from nowhere? Authentic unconditional positive regard and empathic understanding *are* the magic. So:

> *Why be the magician*
> *when you can be the magic?*

Empathic understanding is . . .

Being empathic is demanding – the therapist needs to be strong yet also gentle. To be empathic means to enter the world of another as if it were one's own, yet without ever losing the 'as if' quality. The therapist is flexible, altering, changing, fluid – engaging in a sensitive togetherness as a delicate, confident companion. The therapist may at first 'simply' listen and really hear, and then, through ongoing perception checking, enter what is almost an altered state of consciousness – a reciprocal process for both therapist (from tentative to more confident) and client. The essence of the I–thou relationship is an authentic and respectful striving (and accuracy) to do with sensing and communicating with immediacy (not in one's car on the way home!) one's being attuned to client feelings and meanings, including the unspoken and underlying feelings and meanings of which the client is only dimly aware. The therapist strives with an intense focus to understand clients as they experience themselves to be, from the client's own internal frame of reference (their sensations, perceptions, meanings and memories).

For those who say that client-centred therapy is all about feelings, or too heavily focused on feelings, Rogers stressed the importance of feelings *and meanings* throughout his entire career.

Predictable process and consequences

If the necessary and sufficient client-centred conditions are present, then the power of the actualising tendency will be released. This is an empowering relationship that taps the growth forces within the client, enabling them to be more in touch with their inner psychophysiological flow. It can be said to have an if–then quality. *If* certain conditions are present, *then* a predictable process will follow; *if* the process ensues, *then* predictable outcomes accrue.

Carl Rogers can provide our final summary of the origins and developments of empathic understanding:

> I think at first I realized that it paid to listen carefully, and I gradually realized that I was listening to understand the feelings and the personal meanings. Sometimes people skip that second part – not only listening to the feelings but the personal meaning that experience has for the individual. Then I realized that I was entering into the private, inner world of the individual, trying to sense the exact nature of that inner world and to move around in it freely and maybe sense it from the inside. I realized that empathy also meant being a companion to the person as they search their own experience. Then I began increasingly to trust my own intuitive understanding; sometimes I would want to say things which had no relation to what the client had just said, and yet it seemed to me important to say.
>
> Gradually my understanding of empathy extended to an intuitive capacity for empathy, where I would find something rising in myself that wanted to be said. It might be bizarre. It might be out of context. But I found that if I voiced it, it often rang a bell with the person and opened up all kinds of areas that had been dimly sensed by the client but not really experienced. I don't really understand the workings of intuition. Do I simply pick up nonverbal cues? I don't think that's sufficient to explain it. Somehow there is a way in which the inner core of me relates to the inner core of the other person, and I understand better than my mind understands, better than my brain understands – I'll put it that way. Mind is greater than brain and, somehow, my nonconscious mind understands more than my conscious mind understands, so I'm able to respond to something in this other person that I didn't know I was responding to.
>
> (Rogers and Russell 2002: pp. 284–5)

Empathic understanding is not a technique

Thou shalt not skill!

Having taken a selective journey through some of the origins and developments of empathic understanding in Chapter 1, we now take a reverse angle view in this section. Very often it seems that people (such as Carl Rogers, trainers, trainees, correspondents and authors) have defined empathic understanding, at least in part, through a process of eliminating what it is *not* as much as by defining and celebrating what empathic understanding *is*. Although this may very well be understandable, it has perhaps also been unfortunate in some respects.

This tendency to define empathy by stating what it is not may be understandable for two reasons. The first is the 'everyday habit' of many human beings of describing how they *are* by saying how they *are not*, as in such phrases as 'I'm not feeling so good', 'I don't feel very happy about that' and, when asked how they are, 'Not too bad'. The second reason is more specific to client-centred therapy, in that to some degree the approach was generated through Carl Rogers and others discovering that traditional counselling methods were not satisfactory either to the therapist or to the clients with whom they worked, and so there was a rebellion against 'directive' therapy. We can readily see, for instance, that the early term '*non*-directive' described, in effect, what this type of counselling was not – simply put, it was not directive. Indeed, throughout the development of client-centred therapy (and the person-centred approach), frequent references can be found that reject *doing to* people in favour of *being with* them.

The regrettable element of this is that defining what something *is not* has a rather defensive feel to it when compared with celebrating fully what something *is*. For instance, so many client-centred counselling (or counselling skills) training courses begin with looking at what client-centred therapy is *not* and what the client-centred therapist *does not do* – for example, the therapist does not show shock or surprise, does not praise, support or encourage, does not diagnose or interpret, and so on.

One feature of client-centred therapy is that it is an opportunity for clients to explore and examine their conditions of worth, including the values of others that have been internalised due to a need to be loved, accepted or valued, rather than because they 'feel right' (or are in harmony with 'organismic valuing'). An example of this might be the woman who has come to realise that first she was someone's daughter, then someone's girlfriend, then someone's employee, then someone's wife, then someone's mother, and so on. Eventually her children become more independent, and she realises that her whole life has been spent meeting the needs of or pleasing others. Those were her roles ('keeping everyone happy'), and those roles carried with them values, guidelines and rules about how they should be fulfilled – 'scripts', if you will. There comes a time when although the *roles* may have been fulfilled, the *person* does *not* feel fulfilled, and she wonders, 'What about me?' – usually accompanied by feelings of guilt, shame and embarrassment about even experiencing such a 'selfish' thought. Yet, as if from deep within, there is *something* (often described as a 'voice') that persists with 'What about me?', and that just cannot successfully or permanently be ignored, suppressed or denied. If this message is heard to the extent of actually acting upon it, often another phase is a feeling of liberation – perhaps the client makes what seems to her at the time to be her own free choices, feeling a greater sense of self-assertion. Yet after a while this sense of new-found freedom loses its depth of meaning, because she realises (sometimes gradually, sometimes as a sudden shock) that what she is now doing is the exact opposite of the previous values, guidelines and rules, and if a construction of self is determined in exact opposition to something, then that something retains a central and powerful position. Thus if he used to say 'Buy blue', she now says 'I'll buy red', and somehow *his blue* is still the determinant. In client-centred theoretical terms, the locus of evaluation is still external ('his red', not 'her blue'). Often another phase is that the woman effectively asks herself 'So who on earth am I, really?', or alternatively she states 'I don't know who I am any more'.

Now turning to counselling training, a colleague described facilitating the first day of a counselling diploma course, when trainees had decided to pool their current knowledge. A line was drawn down the middle of a board under the heading 'Client-Centred Counselling', and one column was marked 'The counsellor does' and the other 'The counsellor does not'. The facilitator was writing up what the students were calling out: 'does not praise, does not rescue, does not reassure', and so on (interestingly, the 'does not' column was the starting point). After writing a few entries in the 'does not' column, the facilitator turned to the group and said, 'Why? Why doesn't the client-centred practitioner do these things?'. Following some debate and exploration, the only explanation or reason that trainees could come up with was that this is what they had been *told* (or had learned) on their previous skills course. Returning to the analogy of our female client, if traditional therapies were to be seen as 'his red' it would be most regrettable if client-centred therapy were to be the equivalent of 'her blue' for no other reason than a dislike of or rebellion against 'his red' – yet maybe something akin to this was an understandable developmental phase in the generation of client-centred therapy. It may well be, too, that counsellor trainees who begin to feel *de*-skilled as a consequence of discovering (or being told) that the techniques that they had learned (and had certificated) are no longer praiseworthy might well enter a phase similar to asking 'So who am I, really?' or 'I don't know who I am or how I'm meant to be any more'. Well, one of the central aims of this book is that moving towards an authentically empathic way of being – a way of being that is *you through and through* – is eminently preferable to learning a (relatively impersonal) plethora of skills and techniques.

There is, perhaps, a vital difference between the analogy of the female client and the person who is hoping to become a client-centred therapist. For the client-centred counsellor trainee, it might go something like this: 'My previous skills course tutors taught and told me *red*. Now these diploma facilitators are saying no, not red, *blue* – and furthermore not only is this a higher-level course, but also they can back up *blue* by quoting Carl Rogers, so they must be right'. Yet to jettison or otherwise discard something for which a certificate has been achieved might not come easy. There is a strong argument for neither red nor blue *if they are simply or only the introjected values of others* (be they authors, facilitators or even Carl Rogers), rather than being based on an internal locus of evaluation – *experiencing* first hand what seems to work for you (preferably both as therapist and client). Better a chosen red experienced at first hand than a second-hand introjected (internalised, the value absorbed or taken on from another) blue! Reading a book may indeed be a part of the entire experiencing of a trainee counsellor, yet the message has to be *try it and see*, or, better still, *be it and see*.

While rejecting 'traditional red' was undeniably a significant feature in the development of client-centred therapy, there was also the equally important element of discovery – of looking for and at what seemed to be more meaningfully therapeutic. It is tragic to witness the way of being that was so dear to Carl Rogers reduced to nothing more than the 'blind' introjection of client-centred beliefs, values and technique-oriented practices – not based on personal discovery, experiencing, feeling and meaning, but on the teachings of trainers (that is, an external frame of reference to learners). What might be the qualitative impact if the starting point for client-centred counsellor training were to be the celebration of what client-centred therapy *is* – taking pride and rejoicing in the journey ahead towards becoming a sensitive companion to clients?

You don't know what you've got until you lose it

It was stated earlier that *to some degree* the development of client-centred therapy was a consequence of discarding many traditional beliefs and methods. However, Rogers also built his research activities around looking at what *did* seem to work and what *was* effective (as described in Chapter 1 and Chapter 3 onwards). Let us nevertheless spend time exploring some of the therapist ways of being with clients that did *not* seem to be effective, or which were deemed to be philosophically dehumanising. Can you, for instance, imagine a therapist saying some or all of the following?

> You poor thing. It is perfectly understandable why you feel the way that you do. Still, you can confide in me, your secrets are safe with me. You know that I'll back you all the way, for I'm on your side. You're not alone. Well done! *(You will be rewarded with oodles of attention and compassion if you focus on your feelings.)* Yes, you can do it – it will be okay. You have been badly treated and, you know, another client of mine had a similar experience and . . . And yet I'm glad you're beginning to sort yourself out, it must be really hard. You are most certainly justified in feeling as you do. Don't you think that a sensible course of action might be to . . .? Yes, you could do this; we could work in achievable stages towards . . . Your tears represent feelings of loss at your unresolved grief and you lack the ego strength to fully deal with this right now, so it will clearly take some time before you do have the inner resources – it is as if I were your parent and as if you were my child. If I were you I'd . . . because this is clearly a case of . . . I understand that when you say this you mean that, don't you? When this happened to me I . . .

No, you cannot imagine a therapist saying all of those things, yet if a bet were to be placed on you recognising and being able to imagine *some* counsellors saying *some* of those things *some* of the time, the person placing the wager would not get good odds! Perhaps the above example can be used to further this process of eliminating what empathic understanding is not.

The *intent* of empathic understanding is not the same as *sympathy* – feeling sorry for a client ('you poor thing') – nor is it an attempt at *rescuing* or *normalising* ('it is perfectly understandable and natural that you feel the way you do'). Empathic understanding is not akin to *befriending* ('you can confide in me, your secrets are safe with me'), nor is it about *supporting* ('I'll back you all the way, I'm on your side'), or *meeting client needs* (whatever they may be). Nor is empathy about *praise* ('well done', or an implied 'you'll be rewarded with oodles of attention and compassion if you focus on your feelings' – the latter hardly conveys *unconditional* positive regard), *encouragement* ('you can do it') or *reassurance* ('it will be okay'). Empathic understanding is not the same as *agreement* ('yes, you have been badly treated'), nor is it about making *comparisons* ('another client of mine had a similar experience and , , ,'), nor is it *patronising* ('I'm glad you're beginning to sort yourself out, it must be really hard'). Empathy is not about making *value judgements* ('you are most certainly justified in feeling as you do'), nor does it involve giving *advice* ('a sensible course of action might be to . . .') or *answers* (which are more often than not disempowering). Empathic understanding has nothing to do with *problem solving* ('you could do this . . .'), *goal setting* ('we could work in achievable stages towards . . .') or *having an agenda* or preconceived ideas (although the therapist *will* have preconceived *beliefs* – a philosophy that underpins the therapeutic approach). Empathic understanding is not about *interpreting* ('your tears represent feelings of loss at your unresolved grief . . .'), *diagnosing* ('and you lack the ego strength to fully deal with this right now'), or giving *prognoses* ('it will clearly take some time before you do have the inner resources'), nor is it based on theories of *transference* ('it is as if I were your parent') and/or *counter-transference* ('and it is as if you were my child'). Empathy is not *confrontational* (in the everyday meaning of 'confrontational' as typified by something like 'I understand that when you say this you mean that, don't you?'), and does not include *inappropriate self-disclosure* ('when this happened to me I . . .'), nor is it about the counsellor *knowing best* ('if I were you I'd . . .' or 'this is clearly a case of . . .').

Nor is empathic understanding *all about feelings*.

And nor is empathic understanding concerned with understanding *about*.

On client-centred training programmes, the issues that cause the most initial concern among trainees are usually praise, encouragement, reassurance, support, rescuing and, above all else, *questioning*. There has frequently been an additional confusion between acceptance and agreement, often linked with confrontation as a 'style' (skill or technique) within counselling. Some research evidence (Vincent 1999a) in support of this comes from having modified, expanded and administered (to counselling and counselling skills training groups), over a period of some 18 years, the *Counsellor Attitude Scale* developed by Richard Nelson-Jones and Dr Cecil H Patterson (Nelson-Jones and Patterson 1975). It can be stated through this and other research (see below) that, *inevitably*, acceptance, agreement, challenging, confrontation, diagnosis, encouragement, evaluation, explaining, focusing, interpretation, leading, mirroring, normalising, paraphrasing, praise, probing, prognosis, questioning, reassurance, reflecting, rescuing, responsibility for clients, suggestion, summarising, support, therapist self-disclosure, transference and counter-transference, 'uh-huh', and 'understanding about' have featured as key issues.

When reviewing studies by Julius Seeman (Seeman 1949) and W Snyder (Snyder 1943) of the early days of client-centred counselling, Carl Rogers noted that:

> counsellors used a number of responses involving questioning, inter-preting, reassuring, encouraging, suggesting. Such responses, though always forming a small proportion of the total, would seem to indicate on the counsellor's part a limited confidence in the capacity of the client to understand and cope with his difficulties. The counsellor still felt it necessary at times to take the lead, to explain the client to himself, to be supportive, and to point out what to the counsellor were desirable courses of action.
>
> (Rogers 1951: pp. 30–31)

It is important to stress that tendencies to praise, support and encourage (and so on) are usually well meant, and indeed may well form part of a helping relationship. Thus there is no need for people who experience such impulses to feel 'bad' about themselves. Nevertheless, it is also true to say that the person who *intends* to praise, support and encourage (and so on) has not fully understood or integrated a *client-centred* way of being.

The 'client-centred counsellor does not' list above contains 30 items in all. It might prove helpful to look at these characteristics, now grouped under 13 headings, in an attempt to grasp more clearly what empathy is not.

Acceptance and agreement

Acceptance

> There's . . . a misunderstanding of unconditional positive regard: To care for the client, to prize the client, doesn't mean that you approve of everything the client does; it means a real caring for the essence of the client.
>
> (Rogers and Russell 2002: p. 284)

As we have seen, Stanley Standal, a student working with Carl Rogers in the early days, came to the conclusion that 'acceptance' was a term which was too easily misunderstood. For instance, acceptance is not the same as *agreement* (see below), nor is it the same as *belief* – yet the term *could* be held to mean either (Standal 1954). For example, if person A believes that the earth is flat, person B can *accept* that this is A's *belief*. Person B does not have to *agree* with A, or *accept* that the earth is, in actual fact, flat. In this instance, if person B were to *agree* with person A, or to *accept* person A's *belief* as *fact*, person B would be in a state of incongruence, because they do *not* believe that the earth is flat, and maybe their *agreement* with person A derives from their own needs for positive regard from person A. In this case there is a strong argument for person B engaging in self-awareness and personal growth work if they wish to become a client-centred therapist! Person B's *agreement* would also be based on their own frame of reference – after all, it is person B who is doing the agreeing.

Incidentally, a more socialist critique of 'acceptance' might be that it can be seen as akin to 'accepting your lot' – that acceptance along the lines of 'that's just the way it is' dissipates energy for action (individual or group) through accepting the status quo.

Agreement

Agreement would often seem to be confused with acceptance (as described above). For instance, how often in a counsellor training group have two people been in some form of dispute where person A *disagrees* with person B and is then *accused* by person B of lacking *acceptance*?

In more basic counselling terms, therapist agreement or disagreement would seem to imply a locus of evaluation that is *external* to the client and *internal* to the therapist (or the theory held by that therapist). Very often counsellor trainees seem to think that it is okay (or 'nice' or 'warm' or 'compassionate') to *agree*, yet not okay (or 'nasty' or 'cold' or 'dispassionate') to *disagree*. However, in terms of the power dynamics in the relationship, does not the right to agree also imply the right (or authority) to disagree? Often agreement is verbalised while disagreement is not. Perhaps we can deduce from this that it feels okay (or acceptable) to be 'nice' and 'warm' and 'compassionate', but not to be 'nasty' or 'cold' or 'dispassionate' – despite the power dynamic being exactly the same.

Clearly agreement *and* disagreement involve *value judgements*, usually from either a therapist or a theoretical frame of reference (or both), and as such both agreement and disagreement are directive, potentially manipulative, and generate a power imbalance in the therapeutic relationship.

Agreement, disagreement, non-agreement and collusion

Trainees and supervisees often become concerned that their acceptance will be received by clients as somehow *condoning* or *colluding* with actions or behaviours that the *counsellor*, in private at least, finds unacceptable or even appalling, such as the client who admits aggressive behaviour towards or abuse of a partner, or self-aggressive or abusive acts. This raises a number of issues, not least of which are the congruence of the therapist and the potential consequences in terms of social responsibility and conscience.

Ideally, it could be argued that a wholly non-judgemental therapist will not face such issues. Yet few counsellors, it seems, have escaped grappling with such feelings, thoughts and meanings. If a therapist *does* experience difficulty in 'reality', what then? If the therapist somehow feigns or puts on a show of acceptance when 'really' he or she is anxious about being perceived as colluding with a hurtful behaviour, the therapist is hardly in a state of congruence. Furthermore, many believe that if a therapist 'privately' agrees or disagrees with a client, then the client will sense that approval or disapproval *at some level*, for clients too have a capacity to be empathic ('reciprocal empathy, being in contact'). Some then go on to say that if clients perceive therapist discomfort at some level, then it is probably best for the therapist to self-disclose, as *unspecified* client sensing could potentially be more harmful than transparency and openness. (This theme is explored more fully in Chapter 3 when looking at empathic understanding in relation to congruence.)

Some practitioners and theorists maintain that the therapist accepts *the client* but *not* her or his *behaviour*, which as we have seen in Chapter 1 is not a wholly satisfactory answer. For instance, if being client-centred includes a belief in engaging with *whole* persons, how can one aspect of a person (their behaviour) be separated out as if it does not matter? Surely behaviour is an integral part of the whole person, and a significant part at that? We have also seen in Chapter 1 that acceptance can be seen as a 'there but for the grace of some deity go I' kind of attitude – if a person has *this* experience, then maybe *that* behaviour is a natural and understandable consequence.

Is it, though, possible for a client to sense *non*-agreement, as compared with *agreement* or *disagreement*? Can a therapist 'suspend' *all* judgement, both positive and negative? Might it even be important for a client to actually *sense* non-agreement? For if a client senses therapist agreement, then feelings of collusion or condoning might well be an outcome, and if a client senses therapist disagreement, devalued and worthless feelings might be the result.

Perhaps this can be brought more to life through an illustration. A young boy is referred for counselling because he has begun to cut himself at school. Each time he does so, those around him (mostly the adults, but peers, too) are very concerned, and their caring leads them to try their utmost to find a way of stopping or preventing such self-harming activities. They can 'accept' the young boy as a valuable person for whom they feel compassion, but they find it very difficult indeed to accept (or have compassion for) him physically cutting himself. The therapist is a human being, too, and *of course* does not like to see self-inflicted scars on such a young person – and would most certainly feel uncomfortable at the notion of therapy somehow condoning or colluding with such behaviour. However, the therapist takes a genuine interest in what is going on for the boy. The therapist is *not* trying, overtly or covertly, to *stop* the behaviour. Rather, the therapist is authentically respectful of the behaviour, and is striving to sense the feelings and meanings associated with this self-harm. Striving to engage with the boy as a *whole* person, it becomes clear that within the boy's self-structure are at least three significant aspects, namely a 'perpetrator' (the boy who is cutting himself), a 'victim' (the boy who is being harmed) and some kind of 'observer/ mediator' who watches over and tries to make sense of what is going on.

If the therapist was to be anxious about *colluding with* or *condoning* the self-harm, this would seem to be to do with 'siding with' the perpetrator construct, and maybe with a failure to rescue or protect the victim, too. This is hardly *unconditional* positive regard, for the perpetrator is 'bad' and the victim is worthy of protection (and the observer/mediator would seem to have been somewhat neglected in this equation, too). The boy at first seems surprised (even shocked) that here is someone who is not trying to *prevent* or *correct* an aspect of his behaviour. Rather, here is someone who actually seems to be taking a 'no strings attached' interest in anything and everything that the boy *is* (including what he *does*) – and he seems to be valued as no more or less worthy *whatever* he decides to disclose. The boy even doubts whether this can be true. However, in part as a consequence of this *unconditional* positive regard, the boy gradually becomes free of any need to be defensive, and thus shares more and more of his inner feelings and meanings, slowly moving towards a greater trust in the therapist's acceptance of his *whole being* as genuine. The boy discovers that his inner 'perpetrator' is actually doing its best to keep him safe – for when the boy feels hurt by *others* he experiences not being able to 'handle it', yet he had also discovered that if he inflicted the pain *on himself by himself,* he *could* manage it. Suddenly, it seems, it becomes possible for him to value his inner perpetrator as a part of him that is well meaning, creative, protective and constructive. Had the therapist neglected, ignored, lacked compassion for or disapproved of the boy's inner perpetrator, it is far less likely that *client* self-acceptance would have emerged.

It is so easy – and it seems so tempting – to be 'seduced into naturally' extending all of our compassion to the *victim,* with the consequence that the perpetrator and the observer/mediator are neglected. When this happens, our positive regard is not unconditional, and opportunities for therapeutic movement may well be thwarted. The young boy in this illustration, through a process of being able to own, value, understand and respect himself more fully, changed his own behaviour. No one had to *do* anything – the therapist 'simply' had to strive to *be,* as fully as was possible, the client-centred core conditions.

The boy did the rest.

Challenging and confrontation

Confrontation often appears as a *technique* that is either taught or learned on many counselling skills courses (and, regrettably, on many counselling programmes, too). Indeed, at the time of writing 'confrontation and/or challenging skills' is on the syllabus of at least three major counselling course validating bodies in the UK. At its 'worst', confrontation would seem to assume a hectoring quality, in that the *implementer of the skill* is seemingly determined to get the client to see things as the counsellor does. At its 'best', the user of counselling skills perceives client incongruence, for example, and is determined to confront the client with this observation in order to ensure that the client sees it, too.

Yet is there really anything more 'confrontational' than authentic unconditional positive regard and genuine (and accurate) empathic understanding? For instance, if clients have low self-esteem as a result of their conditions of worth, introjected values, and needs for positive regard (and so on), and the therapist offers unconditional acceptance and empathic understanding of them, then their very self concept is effectively 'challenged' or 'confronted'. However, the crucial differentiating factor here is to do with therapist *intent,* for in genuinely striving to experience and offer acceptance and empathy, the therapist's intent is *simply and only that* – to strive to the best of their ability to experience and offer the fourth and fifth necessary and sufficient conditions from a position of congruence (the third condition).

Study the writings of Carl Rogers and you will find very few references indeed to challenging or confrontation. *Find* a reference and it will be linked with congruence, not empathy. For example, writing about relationships other than therapy (such as partners, sex partners, colleagues, friends, employers and employees), Rogers states that *congruence* is probably the most important of the three core conditions, and that it:

> may involve confrontation and the straightforward expression of personally owned feelings.
>
> (Rogers 1980: p. 160)

It is important to note that Rogers *excluded* counsellor–client relationships from this, and included 'confrontation' within the client-centred core condition of *congruence, not* within empathic understanding.

When it was stated earlier in this chapter that empathic understanding is not about having an agenda or preconceived ideas, yet it might involve preconceived *beliefs*, remember that one fundamental client-centred belief is in the potential for (client) autonomy and self-direction. Client-centred therapists trust in the resources of clients to 'make what they will' of their therapist's authentic striving to experience and offer unconditional positive regard and empathic understanding. However, this is far from a 'couldn't care less' or 'pass the buck' attitude – if counsellors genuinely intend to offer the core conditions, then they are providing an opportunity for therapeutic growth. This is as far as it is possible to be from *setting out with an intent to* 'confront' or 'challenge'.

During some 20 years spent as a trainer of counsellors, I was intrigued as to why trainees would abandon client-centred principles and resort to confronting or challenging their clients, and two main reasons emerged. Either trainee therapists felt that their clients, the process, or they themselves had become 'stuck', or trainees had been influenced by their supervisor (many of whom described themselves as 'person-centred') into importing ways of being that are contrary to client-centred attitudes. Carl Rogers recognised this himself when he said:

> Sometimes people feel that client-centered therapy is good for going only so far, and when you really strike difficult problems you should probably be more confronting or more this or more that. I think – and I feel quite strongly from my experience – that that is really a mistaken line of thought. I think that when the situation is most difficult, that's when a client-centered approach is most needed, and what is needed there is a deepening of the conditions we've talked about – not trying something more technique oriented. It might be worth saying what I've probably said before: in this technological age, an approach that simply lives a philosophy and puts its trust in the capacities of the client seems lacking in glamour, compared to things that try all sorts of tricks and techniques and do different things and try different procedures. It interests me that people who use that sort of an approach often burn out because they just come to the end of their rope; whereas when you get nourishment from the client by seeing the client grow, that's very rewarding.
>
> (Rogers and Russell 2002: pp. 258–9)

Diagnosis, evaluation and prognosis

> The whole diagnostic look at an individual is in sharp contrast to the I–Thou kind of relationship.
>
> (Rogers and Evans: 1975, p. 25)

Therapist diagnosis, evaluation and prognosis clearly do not respect the inner resources of *clients* and their potential and capacity for self-direction, as there is an obvious implication that actually the therapist, not the client, knows best. Carl Rogers wrote that:

If we can provide understanding of the way the client seems to himself at this moment, he can do the rest. The therapist must lay aside his preoccupation with diagnosis and his diagnostic shrewdness, must discard his tendency to make professional evaluations, must cease his endeavors to formulate an accurate prognosis, must give up the temptation subtly to guide the individual, and must concentrate on one purpose only; that of providing deep understanding and acceptance of the attitudes consciously held at this moment by the client as he explores step by step into the dangerous areas which he has been denying to consciousness.

(Rogers 1946: p. 420)

Writing of client-centred principles applied to a learning context, Carl differentiated between empathic understanding and evaluative ways of being, stating of empathy that:

This kind of understanding is sharply different from the usual evaluative understanding, which follows the pattern of 'I understand what is wrong with you'. When there is a sensitive empathy, however, the reaction in the learner follows something of this pattern: 'At last someone understands how it feels and seems to be *me*, without wanting to analyze or judge me. Now I can blossom and grow and learn.'

This attitude of standing in the students' shoes, of viewing the world through their eyes, is almost unheard of in the classroom. But when the teacher responds in a way that makes the students feel *understood* – not judged or evaluated – this has a tremendous impact.

(Rogers 1980: pp. 272–3)

Diagnosis, evaluation and prognosis necessarily involve *judgements*, and being judgemental is not in accord with congruently experiencing and offering both unconditional positive regard and empathic understanding:

Yet it would appear to be true that whether the theme is evaluative or self-concerned, there is slightly less of full respect for the other person than in . . . thoroughly empathic understandings.

(Rogers 1951: p. 45)

If therapists are absorbed with their own processing, or are considering courses of action, then without doubt there is a decreased focus on the world of the client. Even accuracy of evaluation is irrelevant here, because any 'objective' judgement means less respect for client self-direction:

On the other hand, to enter deeply with this man into his confused struggle for selfhood is perhaps the best implementation we now know for indicating the meaning of our basic hypothesis that the individual represents a process which is deeply worthy of respect, both as he is and with regard to his potentialities.

(Rogers 1951: p. 45)

Returning to this theme in 1980, Carl Rogers was able to categorically state that:

Brilliance and diagnostic perceptiveness are unrelated to empathy. It is important to know that the degree to which therapists create an empathic climate is not related to their academic performance or intellectual competence (Bergin and Jasper 1969; Bergin and Solomon 1970). Neither is it related to the accuracy of their perception of individuals or their diagnostic competence. In fact, it may be negatively related to the latter (Fiedler 1953). This is a most important finding. If neither academic brilliance nor diagnostic skill is significant, then clearly an empathic quality belongs in a different realm of discourse from most clinical thinking – psychological and psychiatric. I believe that therapists are reluctant to accept the implications.

> (Rogers 1980: pp. 149–50)

Much of Carl's earlier writing to do with diagnostic evaluation stemmed from his reactions against the psychoanalytic approaches that were so prevalent at the time. For instance, Rogers believed that the diagnostic testing of patients objectifies people rather than prizing them, and thus was 'worse than a waste of time. It is destructive . . .' (Rogers and Evans 1975: p. 98). While Carl Rogers did believe that childhood experience (such as the introjection of values from significant others, culminating in our conditions of worth) is a force to be reckoned with, and therefore that behaviour can be influenced by the past, he added:

> I'm objecting to putting hard-and-fast labels on these processes. I don't like the pigeonholes that Freudian and other theories have promulgated. I think people handicap their thinking when they think in terms of so many labels.
>
> (Rogers and Evans 1975: p. 8)

As we have seen, Rogers went further than simply objecting to labelling when he described targeting individuals in this way as destructive. He added of practitioners who do label:

> I feel that they are destructive, primarily because they make pigeonholed objects out of human beings. If I say you're a paranoid, then you're quite naturally placed. I don't even have to think about you as a person. You belong in that pigeonhole. I've been very interested to see this at work among psychiatrists. If one psychiatrist doesn't like another psychiatrist, then he begins to label him, calls him a manic, or says that he's got paranoid tendencies, or that he's essentially a schizophrenic. They're quite deceptive in that they're really finding a different way of saying they don't like that guy. They have to admit there's some truth in that. Now I think it's a pseudo-thing; I hate pseudo-things. They make it sound as though 'I know what illness you've got'. Physicians overuse labeling, even in physiological diseases; but there are real diseases which they can identify and which deserve a label. To my way of thinking, in psychological states, there are certain patterns. Sure, there are people who are suspicious, and I would call them that instead of giving them a high-falutin label like

paranoid. At any rate, labels give a pseudoscientific sound to what is actually a very loose and unfounded categorization.

(Rogers and Evans 1975: pp. 96–7)

A frequent consequence of diagnostic evaluation was (and often still is) medical prescription, of which Rogers wrote:

Medication is seen so often as a means of dealing with psychotic disorders. Perhaps sometimes that's justified; I don't want to try and step into the field of medicine, but it is most certainly overdone to a great degree. Often patients are medicated in order to be of help to the people caring for them rather than for the welfare of the patient. I think most psychological disorders are psychological in their origin. Their treatment should be dealt with in that fashion.

(Rogers and Evans 1975: pp. 290–91)

Carl believed that much diagnostic testing was *institutionalised*, yet, to further evidence what a useless waste of time such activities are, he pointed out that once a person *leaves* working for 'the establishment' in order to work privately, that practitioner almost never repeats:

[the bureaucratic] rigmarole of diagnoses . . . which shows that he doesn't believe at all in a lot of this folderol he's been sponsoring in the institution. As I see it, rigid classification has no logical or helpful basis. It has just become established as the custom or the tradition, and I wish tradition weren't so hard to change.

(Rogers 1975: pp. 98–9)

Can the client-centred therapist completely do away with diagnosis and evaluation (especially, perhaps, if he or she is working in a medical setting)? This is a vexing question, for even Rogers acknowledged that:

There are difficult border lines, and the border line between what is physical, physiological, medical and illness and what is psychological is sometimes difficult to determine.

(Rogers and Evans 1975: p. 291)

This strongly demonstrates the importance of both supervision and access to medical consultancy.

Carl believed that client *creativity* is generated when people experience freedom from evaluation and measurement from an external locus of evaluation, and wrote that:

Evaluation is always a threat, always creates a need for defensiveness, always means that some portion of experience must be denied to awareness.

(Rogers 1961: p. 357)

If, for example, some aspect of a client is evaluated as 'good' by a therapist, then that makes it all the more difficult for that client to 'admit' (to the therapist or to themselves) that actually they *dislike* this aspect of themselves. Conversely, if a counsellor evaluates some client characteristics as bad, then it makes it all the more difficult for clients to openly express and be those characteristics. Client creativity is fostered through clients moving towards an increasingly inner locus of evaluation.

> It is impossible to be accurately perceptive of another's inner world if you have formed an evaluative opinion of that person. If you doubt this statement, choose someone you know with whom you deeply disagree and who is, in your judgment, definitely wrong or mistaken. Now try to state that individual's views, beliefs and feelings so accurately that he or she will agree that you have sensitively and correctly described his or her stance. I predict that nine times out of ten you will fail, because your judgment of the person's views creeps into your description of them.
>
> (Rogers 1980: p. 154)

Consequently, true empathy is always free of any evaluative or diagnostic quality. The recipient perceives this with some surprise: 'If I am not being judged, perhaps I am not so evil or abnormal as I have thought. Perhaps I don't have to judge myself so harshly.' Thus the possibility of self-acceptance is gradually increased.

None of this means that the therapist becomes some kind of 'cold mirror' – on the contrary, for Carl Rogers differentiated between having a *reaction* and making an *evaluation*. For instance, there is a real contrast between your saying to me 'I am not enjoying reading this book' and 'You are a bad writer'! Your stating to me that you are not enjoying this book leaves me relatively free to keep my own evaluation of my writing, whereas telling me that I am a lousy author condemns me. Note that the same effect would be true of 'I am enjoying reading this book' and 'You are a great writer' – for with the former I remain free to evaluate my own writing, and with the latter the locus of evaluation is effectively taken away from me.

> When the counsellor perceives and accepts the client as he is, when he lays aside all evaluation and enters into the perceptual frame of reference of the client, he frees the client to explore his life and experience anew, frees him to perceive in that experience new meanings and new goals. But is the therapist willing to give the client full freedom as to outcomes? Is he genuinely willing for the client to organize and direct his life? Is he willing for him to choose goals that are social or antisocial, moral or immoral? If not, it seems doubtful that therapy will be a profound experience for the client.
>
> (Rogers 1951: p. 48)

There may well be what might appear to be a conundrum, in that the more accepting the therapist can be of client choice, autonomy and self-direction, the more likely it is that the client will choose healthy, positive directions – the actualising tendency is trustworthy. Carl stated that it could be even more difficult for the therapist to be truly accepting of clients who appear to be 'regressing' rather than growing, to be moving in a direction the therapist believes to be counter to mental well-being – even to be choosing death over life. Yet Rogers wrote that:

> only as the therapist is completely willing that any outcome, any direction, may be chosen – only then does he realize the vital strength

of the capacity and potentiality of the individual for constructive action.

(Rogers 1951: p. 48)

We began this section with a quote from Carl Rogers about diagnosis and evaluation being 'in sharp contrast to the I–Thou kind of relationship'. Let us end this section on a similar, comparative note:

> It was just incredible to have that kind of contact . . . He was a troubled person who was not able to cope with society, that was certain. The one thing that brought him out of it, I feel, was that we were able to form a close person-to-person relationship, and the fact that his feeling about that relationship has continued through eight years is really astonishing. It's even more interesting because, until the very last portion of our contacts together, he would never have openly and consciously admitted that our relationship meant anything to him. It was only by his behavior of continuing to come for interviews that he showed it had a meaning for him. So it's things like that make me feel that if you can reach the psychotic in a real relationship, you've got a chance of bringing him out of his psychosis. I don't underrate the difficulty of reaching such a person as him because, for most individuals who have turned to psychosis as an escape, life has hurt them so much and so many times, and they've been so disappointed in all their personal relationships that they don't believe you. They don't believe you care; they don't believe you're interested; they won't let you reach them because you may hurt them again. We did learn in our research how terribly hard it is to reach some of these people. I still feel that a close human relationship is far more significant than anything doctors with superior knowledge of a patient who is ill can think of doing. I just feel the medical model is ridiculous.
>
> (Rogers and Evans 1975: pp. 95–6)

Explaining, interpreting and normalising

Carl Rogers was keen to distinguish between attempts to *understand* feelings and meanings, and attempts to *explain* or *interpret* them. When writing about group facilitation, for instance, he referred to those facilitators who try to interpret (apparently on behalf of group learning and awareness) that which might not be in conscious awareness, saying that in his experience:

> where leaders have used the technique of interpreting 'unconscious' meanings, such interpretations are usually not facilitating and are frequently disrupting . . . Certainly it is not even justified to say that 'reflecting meanings and intents' is not interpretation in a sense. Nevertheless, there does seem to be a valid distinction between the two, at least in operational terms.
>
> (Rogers 1951: p. 353)

What are these 'operational terms'? Although Rogers grew to dislike the term 'reflection', he differentiated between an attempt to *reflect* feelings and meanings as they appear in the here-and-now awareness of clients, and interpretation, which implies trying to bring 'unconscious' (Carl's quotation marks) experiencing into conscious awareness. He wrote:

> This difference is probably essentially the same as the one that appears to exist between interpretation as used by some psychoanalytic therapists and the method of 'adopting the client's frame of reference' used by client-centred therapists.
>
> (Rogers 1951: p. 354)

Any interpretation of the client by the therapist diminishes the dignity of that client. Carl's reaction against this was a passionate one:

> It made me realize that if I wanted to look like a smart psychologist, I could go ahead and diagnose and advise and interpret. But if I wanted to be effective in working with people, then I might just as well recognize that this person has the capacity to deal with his own problems if I could create a climate where he could do it. Since that time, I would say my whole effort has been focused on the kind of psychological climate that helps the individual to resolve his problems, to develop and to grow.
>
> (Rogers and Evans 1975: p. 27)

'Normalising' is a term that arose in a recent supervision session. The supervisee related how *the counsellor* had *explained* to (or instructed) the client that it was perfectly normal to have the feelings that the client had disclosed. The supervisee seemed somewhat surprised – perhaps *affronted* would be more accurate – that 'normalising' was even worth exploring in supervision, for it was something that had been learned on a client-centred counselling diploma course (and therefore 'normalising' must be 'right'). Yet Carl Rogers quoted the findings of Bergman:

> Evaluation-based and interpretive responses or 'structuring' responses are followed, more often than would be expected by chance, by abandonment of self-exploration.
>
> (Bergman 1951: 216–24)

So how can the *therapist* who has a specific goal *on behalf of* clients, and who thus *explains* something like 'normalcy' to a client in order to achieve that goal, be considered even remotely *client*-centred? Once again, the notion of therapist *intent* is so crucial – there is a huge difference between a client feeling heard, accepted and understood and being *told* that it is normal to have particular feelings.

To the incongruent client and the incongruent therapist, feeling 'stuck' might be accompanied by feelings of discomfort, and the implementation of techniques may well be a defensive reaction aimed at easing such tension. Yet Rogers believed that:

> No approach which relies upon knowledge, upon training, upon the acceptance of something that is *taught*, is of any use. These approaches seem so tempting and direct that I have, in the past, tried a great many of them. It is possible to explain a person to himself, to prescribe steps which should lead him forward, to train him in knowledge about a

more satisfying mode of life. But such methods are, in my experience, futile and inconsequential. The most they can accomplish is some temporary change, which soon disappears, leaving the individual more than ever convinced of his inadequacy.

(Rogers 1961: pp. 32–3)

This reminds me of a client who had received counselling from a predecessor at a medical practice for which I was working. The client began by saying that she had sought help over a bereavement, and that her previous counsellor had been 'fantastic' in the way that she applied techniques and methods (such as writing letters to the deceased, placing them in a box, and then taking them to the park – accompanied by the therapist – to perform a ritual burning). At the time, the client felt truly grateful to her counsellor. Yet some months later (when she arrived to see me), her gratitude had turned to anger and resentment, for she felt as though her previous counsellor had not only taken something away from her (her natural grieving process), but had also left a 'gaping dark space' where her organismic coping methods would have been. In other words, little respect was shown by my predecessor for the potential of this client – her innate tendency to actualise in a constructive way was squashed. What a contrast this is to Rogers saying that:

I think that we do accept the individual *and* his potentiality. I think it's a real question whether we could accept the individual as he is, because often he is in pretty sad shape, if it were not for the fact that we also in some sense realize and recognize his potentiality. I guess I feel, too, that acceptance of the most complete sort, acceptance of this person as he is, is the strongest factor making for change that I know. In other words, I think that it does release change or release potentiality to find that as I am, exactly as I am, I am fully accepted – then I can't help but change. Because then I feel there is no longer any need for defensive barriers, so then what takes over are the forward-moving processes of life itself, I think.

(Rogers 1989: p. 61)

Carl maintained that striving to see a client's world *as that client sees it* is very precious and rare. Yet all too often we instead:

offer another type of understanding which is very different. 'I understand what is wrong with you'; 'I understand what makes you act that way'; or 'I too have experienced your trouble and I reacted very differently'; these are the types of understanding which we usually offer and receive, an evaluative understanding from the outside. But when someone understands how it feels and seems to be *me*, without wanting to analyse me or judge me, then I can blossom and grow in that climate. And research bears out this common observation. When the therapist can grasp the moment-to-moment experiencing which occurs in the inner world of the client as the client sees it and feels it, without losing the separateness of his own identity in this empathic process, then change is likely to occur.

(Rogers 1961: pp. 62–3)

Talking about a demonstration session he had 'performed', Carl spoke about how thoughts about the client occurred to him *after* the session had ended. Such thoughts can always, of course, be the subject of self-reflecting and supervision. *At the time*, though:

> Yesterday's client – I don't remember her exact words – but she said something about how close she felt, and I said we were almost one in this. That's often the feeling that exists, because I'm not trying to think about [how to respond] or interpret, lead, persuade or advise. None of those things are present; I'm just with that client at this moment in exactly the way that he or she is, even though I may not understand what's going on.
>
> (Rogers and Russell 2002: p. 280)

Given the notion (referred to in Chapter 1 and again towards the end of this book) that sociologically, economically and politically there has been a trend, perhaps driven by values more akin to technology than to human beings, to be mechanically problem solving, thereby requiring experts to deliver strategies, tactics, action plans and so on to us, how does this impact upon a client-centred way of being therapeutic with clients? Working in GP surgeries, where there are underlying assumptions based on a medical model of being broken (*ill*) and therefore in need of fixing (a *cure*), patients very often expect their counsellor to be an expert at mending them. Here is a light-hearted caricature:

> Patient: *'My problem is that I am ill, feeling very depressed.'*
> Therapist: *'Perhaps you could tell me more about that . . .'*
> Patient: *'Well, I discovered my partner being unfaithful, I've just been made redundant, I've had test results saying I have an incurable illness, the car packed up the day after the warranty expired, my house burned down . . . oh, and the dog was run over.'*

We might laugh – yet I have seen patient after patient who regard their *problem* as being depression, when in fact they really would be 'nuts' if they were *not* feeling incredibly low (and very often there is a catalogue of tragedies, not just one). Yet they are convinced that they *must* be ill, for they have a prescription from their GP for antidepressants, and surely their doctor would not be prescribing drug treatment if there was no illness to cure. Worse still, there is an expectation that in being referred to see me, they will meet an expert who can help to fix their ailment.

So the temptation to 'normalise' or explain to patients that they are not actually ill can be huge, yet if I do so, I am putting myself in the role of expert, thereby diminishing any trust in the personal resources of clients, and possibly colluding with values internalised into the client's self-concept about being inadequate (for instance, 'I should be able to cope'). My intent in such situations is to be as close to the therapist conditions as I can be, relying on the client to receive these conditions and move with them. If, for instance, a client meets with congruent therapist unconditional positive regard (perhaps a calm acceptance, without judgement, of who and how they are) and empathic understanding, it has been my experience that they themselves will very quickly come to the conclusion that they have every right to feel depressed, and that their feelings and thoughts are worth the effort of understanding and accepting, rather than failings to be fought.

Encouragement, rescuing, support and responsibility

Encouragement

You may recall from earlier on that *encouraging*:

> would seem to indicate on the counsellor's part a limited confidence in the capacity of the client to understand and cope with his difficulties.
> (Rogers 1951: pp. 30–31)

At a fairly mundane level, encouraging a client to pursue a particular course of action (maybe typified by such statements as 'you could have much to gain by approaching this person and talking it through with them' or maybe the more indirectly implied 'have you talked with . . .?') can easily be demonstrated as not being in harmony with client-centred beliefs. The client is being encouraged, directly or indirectly, to take a course of action that the *therapist* thinks is desirable – and there is little respect shown for the inner resources of the client.

Perhaps there is something, too, about actions that seem on the face of it to be *positive*, and those that seem *negative*. A great many trainee counsellors, when asked whether or not it is acceptable to *discourage* a client, would instantly reply that it is blatantly *not* acceptable to discourage. Yet the same trainee may feel far less strongly about *encouraging*. However, just as with *agreement* and *disagreement*, surely the right to do one implies the right to do the other? The power imbalance in the relationship is skewed (that is, primarily with the therapist, not the client) whether encouragement or discouragement is the factor. The trainee counsellor who encourages clients yet baulks at the idea of discouraging them may well *withhold* encouragement at times, rather than actively discouraging – the relationship still remains conditional and imbalanced. Clearly both encouragement and discouragement involve value judgements, and judgements of this kind clearly do not communicate unconditional positive regard and empathic understanding.

Having stated earlier that empathy is *not all about feelings*, all too often, it seems, in the early days of learning the clients of trainees appear to be encouraged to focus almost solely on their feelings, often at the expense of content, thought, behaviours, meanings or memories (as they influence the here and now). Indeed, being 'heady' or cognitive often seems to be frowned upon – and as we have seen, specious arguments about accepting a person yet not that person's behaviour are often utilised in an attempt to justify this. At this perhaps more subtle level, if the therapist consistently responds to disclosures of feelings and not to thoughts, meanings, behaviour or content, then clients are effectively being *encouraged* (or *manipulated* or *directed*) to 'operate' at a feeling level if they are to gain the attention and respect of, and feel valued by, their therapist. Such *therapist* direction cannot be described as *client*-centred.

Rescuing

Rescuing, as with many of the qualities in this section, may also come from an honourable, humane and understandable place although, as with other such characteristics, that 'place' is likely to reside within the *therapist*, not the client. Once again a *judgement* is involved – that the client is worthy of rescuing or needs to be rescued. In this instance there is a lack of respect for the client's own inner resources, and in addition the therapist might be encouraging, creating or promoting dependency. In rescuing a client, the therapist may in effect be colluding with client denials and/or distortions, colluding with the perpetuation of a self-concept that includes the personal construct of being in need of rescue.

At a fundamental level, the counsellor may be colluding with the thwarting of a client's actualising tendency.

Support

Support is not something that the client-centred therapist *intends* to offer to clients. Carl Rogers stated of client-centred therapy:

> It is experienced as basically supporting, but it is in no way supportive. The client does not feel that someone is behind him, that someone approves of him.

> (Rogers 1951: p. 209)

People often respond with not a little scepticism to the statement that client-centred therapists do not intend to be supportive, for how could a therapist be so cold and uncaring yet describe their approach as client-centred? Yet if the therapist sets out to support clients, a judgement has been made – no matter how humane or caring. This judgement is that the client is worthy of (and maybe in need of) the support of the therapist. The therapist has the power to *withdraw* or *withhold* support, and may even be in danger of fostering dependency. Is offering support in keeping with beliefs about client autonomy and self-direction? The answer is no. Is offering support in keeping with beliefs about the inner strengths and resources derived from the actualising tendency? Again the answer is no.

So client-centred therapists do not *intend* to offer support to clients, but rather their *intent* is to strive to both experience and offer authentic unconditional positive regard and empathic understanding. Clients may well experience, at times at least, this genuine offering of respect and empathy *as supportive*. However, that is up to *clients* to experience and decide. The therapist *intent* remains fundamental – to offer certain conditions which it is believed are not only necessary but also sufficient to create a relationship within which there is the potential for therapeutic growth.

Responsible to and not for

The notion that therapists are responsible *to* clients but not *for* them frequently arises in counsellor training programmes, and links with what Carl Rogers meant when he wrote of the 'basic struggle' of the counsellor:

> only when the counsellor, through one means or another, has settled within himself the hypothesis upon which he will act, can he be of

maximum aid to the individual. It has also been my experience that the more deeply he relies upon the strength and potentiality of the client, the more deeply does he discover that strength.

(Rogers 1951: p. 48)

In much the same way as John Shlien wrote that 'undeserved denigration of the technique (of reflecting) leads to fatuous alternatives in the name of congruence' (Shlien 1986), so too can the idea of responsible *to* but not *for* be misunderstood or even abused. Imagine two people, A and B, in relationship. Throughout the relationship A is critical of B, constantly and incessantly knowing best, putting B down, saying that B is wrong, is no good, and so on. B eventually discovers the resources to voice a dislike of A's 'superior' way of being, only to hear from A that *B* is wholly responsible for what B feels, for 'no one can *make* B feel anything'. This is an utter cop-out! Sometimes even an utter cop-out, an attempt at the abdication of responsibility such as this, can mistakenly be 'justified' in the name of congruence. Why 'mistakenly'? Because in this instance, unconditional positive regard and empathic understanding are clearly not integrated and deeply held beliefs that guide A's way of being. At the same time, if therapists are without influence, why be a therapist? Perhaps it would be more accurate to say that client-centred therapists need to be responsible *to and for themselves,* and responsible *to* but *not for* their clients. And therapists being responsible *to and for* themselves *includes* integrated and deeply held beliefs and attitudes that underpin a disciplined client-centred way of being:

> It would appear that for me, as counsellor, to focus my whole attention and effort upon understanding and perceiving as the client perceives and understands, is a striking operational demonstration of the belief I have in the worth and the significance of this individual client. Clearly the most important value which I hold is, as indicated by my attitudes and my verbal behaviour, the client himself. Also the fact that I permit the outcome to rest upon this deep understanding is probably the most vital operational evidence which could be given that I have confidence in the potentiality of the individual for constructive change and development in the direction of a more full and satisfying life. As a seriously disturbed client wrestles with his utter inability to make any choice, or another client struggles with his strong urges to commit suicide, the fact that I enter with deep understanding into the desperate feelings that exist but do not attempt to take over responsibility, is a most meaningful expression of basic confidence in the forward-moving tendencies in the human organism.

(Rogers 1951: pp. 35–6)

When might a therapist struggle with the notion of not being responsible *for* a client? Other than with malpractice, the most difficult moments would seem to be when there is a considerable risk or danger, either to or from the client. Carl said that therapists need to ask themselves just how far their respect for clients actually goes. Can the therapist, for instance, maintain a deep respect for the capacity of individuals when life is literally at stake? If therapists are reaching or have reached the end of their capacity to experience and offer unconditional acceptance and respect, what are the consequences then? Rogers wrote that:

One would be the hypothesis that 'I can be successfully responsible for the life of another'. Still another is the hypothesis 'I can be temporarily responsible for the life of another without damaging the capacity for self-determination'. Still another is 'The individual cannot be responsible for himself, nor can I be responsible for him, but it is possible to find someone who can be responsible for him'.

(Rogers 1951: p. 47)

Thus one scenario might be that there are those therapists who believe that they *can* be (or even *are*) responsible for the lives of others, namely their clients. Another example might be therapists who believe that neither they nor their clients are *able to* (or *should*) take responsibility, in which case the client might either be referred to someone from the first extreme, or the client might somehow end up being cast adrift. Yet a third possibility is the therapist who tries to *temporarily* set aside client-centred beliefs in the fundamental trustworthiness of the actualising tendency, believing that client autonomy can be restored to them once this 'blip' has passed. Carl Rogers questioned what the crucial factor might be in all of this – is it communication from a frame of reference external to the client (such as therapists voicing that they are willing to continue seeing the client, or communicating a belief in the client's ability to choose, or referring the client to another resource), or is it holding the client in deep respect, whether indicated from the internal or external frame of reference? Rogers entered the moral and ethical debate as to whether the counsellor has the authority to permit clients to seriously consider suicide or psychosis without making a positive effort to prevent or circumvent such choices, asking whether not making such an effort is an abdication of our general social responsibility. He concluded that:

these are deep issues, which strike to the very core of therapy. They are not issues which one person can decide for another. Different therapeutic orientations have acted upon different hypotheses. All that one person can do is to describe his own experience and the evidence which grows out of that experience.

(Rogers 1951: p. 48)

And that is precisely what Carl Rogers did. In his formulation of the necessary and sufficient conditions, he placed unconditional positive regard *before* empathic understanding, believing that empathy is the primary vehicle for communicating our deep respect for the actualising tendency:

We might say, then, that for many therapists functioning from a client-centred orientation, the sincere aim of getting 'within' the attitudes of the client, of entering the client's internal frame of reference, is the most complete implementation which has thus far been formulated for the central hypothesis of respect for and reliance upon the capacity of the person.

(Rogers 1951: p. 36)

It would seem, then, that it is vital for client-centred therapists to explore the limits to which they are prepared to go within this philosophy, to determine just how strong their belief in the right of clients to self-determination actually is. It could even be posited that the more exceptions there are to unconditional positive regard, the less client-centred and therapeutic the relationship will be. And this feels really, really tough – for having established that it is in no way client-centred to *rescue*, nor could it be described as compassionate to stand idly by watching someone drown. Taking responsibility for the thrashing client might involve diving in the water and dragging them to the safety of dry land – yet what if the client somehow *needed* to flail prior to treading water? Perhaps worse still, what if the client really, truly, deeply wanted to drown? Could the therapist sleep at night knowing that the client could have been saved? Abdication of respons-ibility might involve referring to a lifeguard – the therapist is unable to help, clients cannot help themselves, so there is no option other than to refer to a third party who can help. Then again, the sinking client could be thrown a lifeline by the therapist – the client can learn to swim at a later date, once they have been saved. These are real issues – you cannot counsel a cadaver. When writing of person-centred group work, Rogers stated that one obligation of the facilitator was to define the limits within which unconditional positive regard could be offered. Perhaps the same obligation could be said to hold true for the client-centred therapist.

Clearly there are some deep and, to many, troublesome issues surrounding the extent to which beliefs in unconditional positive regard and the right of clients to self-determination can be lived out – matters of personal and social conscience. What a difference there can be between a philosophical classroom debate and losing a client through suicide. Yet let us not forget the paradox, too – the more the actualising tendency is trusted, the more experience of its trustworthiness there tends to be.

Focusing, leading and suggestion

Focusing

Some fine distinctions need to be made when looking at the issues that surround focusing. If it is the *therapist* who decides what is meaningful to focus upon, then clearly the *therapist* is leading (see below), and this could not be deemed to be client-centred. However, most therapist communications involve a *choice* on the part of the therapist, as client disclosures very often involve many feelings and meanings and/or potential sensations and meanings, and rarely can the therapist effectively capture all of them in one verbalisation. To attempt to communicate *all* feelings and meanings (and all *potential* feelings and meanings) can become somewhat clumsy or cumbersome, or the therapist might be trying too hard to 'get it right' (maybe connected with their own conditions of worth), and so on. So what does guide therapists with regard to communicating their sensing of different aspects of client disclosures? Perhaps a fairly basic paraverbal commun-ication exercise might illustrate this ('paraverbal' means the *way* we speak, rather than *what* is spoken; it includes volume, speed, pitch, and so on). Consider the following statement:

I never said he stole that money.

Imagine saying the above sentence placing the stress on the word 'I', and the meaning becomes *I didn't say anything, but someone else did*. Place the stress on the word 'never' and it becomes *a protestation of innocence*. Place the stress on 'said' and there is *a belief but not a verbalisation.* Stress 'he' and *the accusation is levelled at a different person.* Stress 'stole' and the meaning might become *borrowed.* Stress 'that' and *it was different money that he stole.* Stress 'money' and *the theft was of something different.* Thus this sentence, consisting of just seven words, can have at least seven *different* meanings depending upon the paraverbal nature of the way it is spoken. The therapist who communicates a sense of righteous indignation because the word 'never' was stressed by the client is closer to empathic understanding than the therapist who picks up on theft because his or her own house was burgled last week! In stressing the importance of paraverbal communication, Rogers wrote that:

> even the transcripts of our recorded cases may give to the reader a totally erroneous notion of the sort of relationship which existed. By persistently reading the counselor responses with the wrong inflection, it is possible to distort the whole picture.
>
> (Rogers 1951: pp. 27–8)

The same kind of deliberation also applies to *non-verbal* communication – the client might make significant eye contact when speaking a particular word, or grimace, or tense a part of their body. If 'focusing' in this way is based on what seems significant *to* the client, *from* the client, then it could well be seen as part of being client-centred. If focusing is based on anything other than what seems significant to the client (that is, it is significant to the therapist, or psychological theory, for instance), then it is not client-centred.

Incidentally, a further development has been that some theorists and practitioners regard 'focusing' as meaning that therapists focus primarily upon themselves. Carl Rogers clearly wished to distance himself from this view, in that while it is true that therapist congruence is a core condition for client-centred therapy, it is fundamentally to do with embodying authentic unconditional positive regard and empathic understanding – and the more that therapists become absorbed with themselves (*'therapist*-centred therapy'!), the less attention is available for clients. For therapists to internally monitor themselves along the lines of 'How am I experiencing myself in relation to and in relationship with this client?' seems fair enough in terms of striving to be congruent, and especially if the aim of such self-awareness is to access, maintain and enhance the degree of unconditional positive regard and empathic understanding that the therapist is able to give to the therapeutic relationship. However, if the focus of the therapy was to shift too far away from the client because the therapist is so self-absorbed and self-monitoring, then that relationship would lose client-centred therapeutic integrity.

Leading and suggestion

Issues about leading and suggestion bear many similarities to the reasoning outlined above for *non-acceptance, evaluation* and *rescuing.* Something that Carl Rogers wrote about person-centred group facilitation can be reapplied to client-centred therapy:

> What the facilitator does *not* do is perhaps as important as what he or she does do. A facilitator committed to a person-centered way of being does not guide, push or prod. He or she is content to go with the

process of the group, whether rapid or slow. He or she does not persuade or take sides. The facilitator does not offer solutions. His or her basic trust is in the wisdom which, from experience, he knows resides in the group, if he can only create the psychological climate in which it can emerge.

(Rogers and Ryback 1984: p. 6)

Put simply and briefly, client-centred therapy is about the therapist either following or 'tracking' clients, or being alongside clients (as a respectful and sensitive companion) in their journeys of self-discovery. *If* the *therapist* leads (other than occasionally voicing a perception of which the client is as yet only dimly aware), *then* the relationship *cannot* be client-centred. If any suggestion comes from a frame of reference that is *external* to the client, the therapy cannot be client-centred.

A brief journey into power

Most procedures in psychotherapy may be placed on a scale having to do with power and control. At one end of the scale stand orthodox Freudians and orthodox behaviorists, believing in a politics of author-itarian or elitist control of persons 'for their own good', either to produce better adjustment to the status quo or happiness or content-ment or productivity or all of these. In the middle are most of the contemporary schools of psychotherapy, confused, ambiguous or paternalistic in the politics of their relationships (though they may be very clear regarding their therapeutic strategies). At the other end of the scale is the client-centered, experiential, person-centered approach, consistently stressing the capacity and autonomy of the person, her right to choose the directions she will move in her behavior, and her ultimate responsibility for herself in the therapeutic relationship, with the therapist's person playing a real but primarily catalytic part in that relationship.

(Rogers 1978: pp. 20–1)

Let us temporarily step out of *'Thou Shalt Not Skill'* to look at the notion of power and control, for many of the attitudes and practices rejected by Carl Rogers link with beliefs about the location of power and control in psychotherapy. Carl said that elements we might explore include:

Who will be controlled? Who will exercise control? What type of control will be exercised? Most important of all, toward what end or what purpose, or in the pursuit of what value will control be exercised?

(Rogers and Evans 1975: p. lxii)

Therapists, said Rogers, first need to think about both their general and their specific goals when practising therapy, to settle within themselves their purpose in being therapists in the first place. Although he agreed with the prevailing scientific view that research can help us to determine the means of achieving the goals that we have settled upon, Rogers also thought that the tradition had been for an individual or group (such as a therapeutic approach) to gain the power to use their methods. Individuals are then exposed to these established conditions and there is a high probability that outcomes will be in line with them, leading to an ongoing, socialised organisation that continues to produce the desired behaviour in patients or clients. He believed, with regard to the first point, that:

> It is possible for us to choose to value man as a self-actualizing process of becoming; to value creativity, and the process by which knowledge becomes self-transcending.
>
> (Rogers and Evans 1975: p. lxxviii)

Client-centred therapist conditions can be set with a *minimum* of power or control, and client outcomes are to do with self-actualising, a process whereby clients move towards greater self-responsibility:

> Thus such an initial choice would inaugurate the beginnings of a social system or subsystem in which values, knowledge, adaptive skills, and even the concept of science would be continually changing and self-transcending. The emphasis would be upon man as a process of becoming.
>
> (Rogers and Evans 1975: p. lxxix)

Not only do therapists establish the conditions in which they work, but also clients give power to therapists:

> The client, a somewhat lost, confused, not too well-ordered person, has typically never met anyone with such a powerfully directed focus and lived belief. As already indicated, the client's position as a failed person hoping to find his way also lends substance to the therapist's power.
>
> (Barton 1974: p. 191)

And therapist power has a value base that the therapist cannot but help communicate:

> The methods the therapist uses . . . represent values. They communicate the essential therapeutic values . . . or the lack of them. The therapist's methods are not simply objective techniques but are part of the therapist as a person. The therapist as a person relates to the client as a person. The responses of the therapist reveal what the therapist values. These responses also reveal whether the therapist considers himself or herself an expert by leading, questioning, interpreting, guiding, suggesting, advising, or whether the therapist places the responsibility on the client by . . .
>
> (Patterson 2000: p. 121)

Many trainee therapists have said that their main reason for wanting to become a client-centred therapist is their *desire to be of help* (wanting either to 'give something back' to repay valued help that they themselves received, or to offer to others the assistance they themselves never received) – yet Carl Rogers believed that even this ideal or goal was somewhat secondary, for:

in the most real moments of therapy I don't believe that this intention to help is any more than a substratum on my part . . . Surely I wouldn't be doing this work if it wasn't part of my intention. And when I first see the client that's what I hope I will be able to do, is to be able to help him. And yet in the interchange of the moment, I don't think my mind is filled with the thought of 'now I want to help you'. It is much more 'I want to understand you. What person are you behind that paranoid screen, or behind all these schizophrenic confusions, or behind all these masks that you wear? In your real life, who are you?'. It seems to me that is a desire to meet a person, not 'now I want to help'. It seems to me that I've learned through my experience that when we can meet, then help does occur, but that's a by-product.

(Rogers 1989: p. 55)

Let us now return to the *'Shalt Nots'* of meeting with a valued client.

Mirroring, paraphrasing, reflecting and summarising

Let one thing be absolutely clear:

There is no such thing as a client-centred skill.

Likewise, Carl Rogers wrote of therapist communicating that:

If it is simply reflection, that's no good. That's just a technique. It must be a desire to understand empathically, to really stand in the client's shoes and to see the world from his vantage point.

(Rogers and Evans 1975: p. 29)

Many people react with astonishment to the statement that *there is no such thing as a client-centred skill*, yet we have seen in Chapter 1 how Carl was *appalled* at the way in which client-centred therapy (and empathic understanding in particular) had become a caricature of itself, and he was utterly dismayed at the way in which in many counsellor training programmes the learning or teaching of 'wooden techniques' had somehow replaced *becoming a person*, and *developing a client-centred way of being*.

It is clear that, in part, techniques such as mirroring, paraphrasing, reflecting and summarising became associated with client-centred therapy because they are relatively 'non-directive' when compared with more overtly manipulative practices (to give an extreme example, paraphrasing a client's words is less directive than referring a client for electroconvulsive treatment). It is also true (and by his own admission), that *in the early days* of developing client-centred therapy, Carl Rogers and his colleagues *did* pay considerable attention to therapist techniques. It may be, too, that those who desire to be of help to others readily grasp skills and techniques that are relatively easily taught or learned.

Approaching this from a different angle, surely *a skill is a skill is a skill* whatever the orientation of the therapist? If, for instance, a transactional analyst mirrors or reflects something that a client has said, does it mean that for that moment only the therapist is suddenly 'being client-centred'? If a psychodynamic practitioner paraphrases a client disclosure, has that analyst suddenly ceased to become psychodynamic and miraculously converted to being client-centred? If a cognitive–behavioural therapist summarises what the client has just shared, has that therapist somehow 'integrated' client-centredness into cognitive–behavioural therapy? The answer to all of these questions is *of course not*. In part we can say 'of course not' because Rogers stated that the six client-centred conditions of contact, client incongruence, therapist congruence, unconditional positive regard and empathic understanding, and client perception of the therapist's respect and empathy were both necessary *and sufficient* – and that the 'importing' of elements from other therapies goes a long way towards *destroying* the possibilities for a therapeutic encounter. And in part we can assert 'of course not' because a reflection is a reflection *whatever* the therapeutic approach of the therapist (indeed, such communication skills have even been adopted to enhance sales techniques and other forms of 'people management'). So let it be repeated, *there is no such thing as a specifically client-centred skill*.

To *paraphrase* or *summarise* what a client has just said, the practitioner needs to develop a fairly good memory that includes the ability to absorb, store and recall information, have a reasonable vocabulary and understanding of the language being spoken (including synonyms), and have the ability to re-order words (usually into a more succinct form) without losing their essential meaning. While this may, then, involve a degree of cleverness (and indeed may form the basis of a helpful relationship), it does not necessarily have to involve the demanding task of truly and delicately entering the world of another and striving to respectfully experience and understand it as the other person experiences it, including their feelings, meanings and memories. Paraphrasing or summarising hardly represents an attempt to communicate the fruits of a counsellor having strived to sensitively and delicately enter the world of another and to respectfully experience and understand it as the other person experiences and understands it.

Another way of seeing how client-centred therapy is more to do with an empathic way of being than with the implementation of skills might be to look at the technique called 'reflecting' – and 'reflecting' or 'reflecting feelings' appear on the curriculum of the majority of counselling skills and even (allegedly) client-centred counsellor training programmes. Yet Carl Rogers wrote of the influence of a Rankian trained practitioner:

> The next social worker that I employed in Rochester was Elizabeth Davis . . . and one of the things she taught me was to focus on the feelings that were being expressed and to respond to those feelings. It was this that led to this whole idea of reflection of feelings, which is much misunderstood.
>
> (Rogers and Russell 2002: p. 113)

Although Carl expressed gratitude for this having improved his work early in his career, he later wrote of '*reflect* becoming in time a word that made me cringe' (Rogers 1980: p. 138). It is possible to reach the conclusion from Carl's words that the learning of reflecting skills (or the technique of 'reflecting feelings') *could* therefore be a useful step on the way towards developing an empathic way of being. That may be – yet imagine the counselling *skills* trainee who has received positive feedback and indeed certification for both open-ended questioning and reflecting discovering later (when training to become a client-centred *therapist*) that not only is there nothing specifically client-centred about the generic skill of reflecting, but also Rogers 'cringed' at the notion. Worse still, if the implementer of the skill of reflecting primarily focuses on *feelings*, the relationship comes to have a narrow focus, as the therapist is not engaging with a *whole* person – it becomes *directive* (the *client* is not leading) and *judgemental* – and the client's world of personal meanings, thoughts, behaviours and memories may be neglected.

To illustrate this point, if another person is speaking, it is not too difficult for listeners to train themselves to listen for key words or phrases and to 'reflect them back' to the speaker. However, this is largely an exercise in discerning listening, memory and recall – the listener does not need to invest their whole being in this exercise, as it is primarily their intellect that is utilised. For instance, it is possible to reflect a client's words with little or no compassion or caring. Indeed, one could listen for and reflect the key words or phrases of someone speaking on television, or from a passage in a book. There is no necessity for many of the necessary or sufficient conditions – there is no absolute need for 'psychological contact' or a quality of presence, no essential requirement for the listener to be congruent, no necessity for great respect for the inner world of client feelings and meanings (if engaged in a primarily intellectual exercise), and no real demonstration of empathy or understanding. Instead, this could be a demonstration of competency in hearing and recall. Hence Rogers wrote that he had become more and more 'allergic' to the use of the term 'reflecting'.

However, Carl Rogers did acknowledge that viewing or listening to his demonstration counselling interviews could easily result in the idea that he did regularly 'reflect'. It was a friend and former colleague of his, Dr John Shlien, who wrote to Rogers that 'reflection is unfairly damned', for while Shlien agreed with him that reflecting purely as a technique or skill lacked quality of presence, Shlien also maintained that reflecting can be 'an instrument of artistic virtuosity in the hands of a sincere, intelligent, empathic listener' and that 'it made possible the development of client-centred therapy, when the philosophy alone could not have. Undeserved denigration of the technique leads to fatuous alternatives in the name of congruence' (Rogers 1986: pp. 375–7).

This correspondence with John Shlien enabled Carl to further clarify his process of communicating empathy. Rogers was *not* trying to 'reflect feelings' but *was* engaged in a process more akin to *'perception checking'* – by which he meant a cautious (or tentative) offering of his sensing of what the client was experiencing from moment to moment, and being constantly prepared to amend his sensing in response to client feedback. At the same time, Rogers acknowledged that there was a sense in which the therapist is 'holding up a mirror' to the client, a 'mirror' that enables clients to see and experience themselves more clearly. Carl stated that Sylvia Slack expressed this 'beautifully' when she wrote:

> It was like Dr Rogers was a magical mirror. The process involved my sending rays toward that mirror. I looked into the mirror to get a glimpse of the reality that I am. If I had sensed the mirror was affected by the rays being received, the reflection would have seemed distorted and not to be trusted. Although I was aware of sending rays, their nature was not truly discernible until they were reflected and clarified by the mirror. There was a curiosity about the rays and what they revealed about me. This experience allowed me an opportunity to get a

view of myself that was untainted by the perceptions of outside viewers. This inner knowledge of myself enabled me to make choices more suited to the person who lives within me.

(Slack 1985: pp. 35–42)

Thus therapist communications need to be undistorted, and that means not 'polluting' the internal frame of reference of the client.

Watching videos of Carl Rogers in action has been experienced as confusing by some viewers. In one session, for instance, Rogers seemed almost to repeat, word for word, what the client had just said. However, in the question-and-answer session that followed the demonstration, he explained that in *that* moment, with *that* particular client, using the client's own words and speaking in the first person (as if he were that client) seemed the best way to try to enter her frame of reference, her world of feelings and personal meanings. In other demonstration therapy sessions, Carl was perceived quite differently, so we can see that striving to empathically understand another is far from being a 'wooden', 'cold' or systematic technique. Rather, empathy is a fluid yet consistent way of being with another, that will vary from client to client and with the same client over time (from, for instance, tentative to more confident, as we saw in Chapter 1). In an interview given just months prior to his death (transcription published posthumously in 2002), Carl Rogers said:

> It is interesting that the term *reflection of feelings* still is a current issue . . . When one looks at it from an external point of view, and studies a transcript of an interview, for example, it is quite clear that the therapist very often is giving a restatement, a fresh verbal organization of the feelings and personal meanings the client has expressed. In that sense, reflection of feelings seems like a fairly accurate term. But from the point of view of the therapist, when good therapy is going on, the therapist is not trying to reflect feelings. He is trying to check under-standings or test perceptions. He's trying to say, 'Is this the way it is in you? Am I getting the flow of your feeling? Am I understanding the nuances of what's going on in you? Are you saying that you're angry with your father?' Although those questions as I'm now stating them are usually not verbalized, that's always the intent.

(Rogers and Russell 2002: pp. 253–4)

Praise and reassurance

Praise

Many people over the years have expressed how, without praise, their learning would have been impaired in some way, or that if only they had received more positive feedback they would have done better. Praise is often viewed as a human need, and as a very good thing indeed.

Once again, though, praising involves the *judgement* that something *merits* positive feedback. Does the counsellor feel the same way about voicing criticism or negative feedback to clients? If the counsellor does *not* feel the same way, how can it be argued that therapist positive regard is *unconditional*? For sure, if therapists grant themselves the power and authority to praise and encourage and support and reassure, then by implication they also grant themselves the power and authority to chastise or criticise, or at the very least to withhold or withdraw praise, encouragement, reassurance and other apparently 'positive' feedback.

Empathic understanding is about entering the *internal* frame of reference of the other. Praise indicates that the *therapist* believes that the other person is deserving of positive feedback – from a locus of evaluation *external* to the client. Lest it again be thought that the client-centred therapist lacks warmth, if a client clearly feels good about themselves or something they have achieved, and the therapist empathically understands this *from within the client's frame of reference* – and the client perceives this appreciation – then that relationship will not lack warmth. Rather, being in tune with the client's internal locus of evaluation, it will have deeper and more personal meanings for that client.

Reassurance

Again, recall the words of Carl Rogers:

> reassuring . . . would seem to indicate on the counsellor's part a limited confidence in the capacity of the client to understand and cope with his difficulties. The counsellor still felt it necessary at times to take the lead . . .
>
> (Rogers 1951: pp. 30–1)

Reassurance, at least in the early days of counsellor training, is often seen as another of those 'nice' qualities. Without intending any disrespect for the word 'nice', can we nevertheless examine the concept of 'nice' in a client-centred therapist and client context?

First, let us question where the *need* to reassure comes from. If it is the *therapist's* need to reassure, then no matter how honourable or nice a place that need comes from, it is clearly the *therapist's* need, and *not* the need of the client, and so it can hardly be described as *client*-centred. Alternatively, the therapist might sense a need for reassurance coming from the client, and there are those who see counselling as being about responding to or meeting such needs. At first glance, this might even seem to make some sense, yet it does not stand up to more serious scrutiny.

The statement that client-centred therapy is not at all to do with meeting client needs often meets with surprise. Yet ask yourself 'If a client expresses the need for me to provide all the answers and solutions, is to do so client-centred?' The consensus of opinion would surely be that client-centred therapy is *not* about the therapist providing solutions, so in this instance responding to an expressed client need by simply going along with it would clearly be inappropriate. The client-centred therapist might well strive to respect and empathically understand a client's needs, but that is not the same as *judging* the need as okay or not okay (from a frame of reference *external* to that client) and responding accordingly. Another question could be asked: 'What if it is a client need to seriously abuse the therapist in some way?'. Does the therapist creating a 'permissive' atmosphere mean that counsellors respond to client needs by becoming their victim? Of course not! If it is clear that there are some client needs that a therapist would certainly *not* meet, who determines which needs it might be okay for the therapist to meet? If the *therapist* determines what is and is not acceptable, then 'say goodbye' to *unconditional* positive regard. If the *client* determines what needs the therapist will meet, 'say goodbye' to *therapist* positive self-regard! Client-centred practice is about authentically and unconditionally *respecting* all client needs – the therapist 'responds' to such needs not by trying to meet them, but by striving to sense and understand the feelings and personal meanings that generate such needs.

Thus responding to client needs has no place whatsoever in client-centred therapy. Whatever the context, *reassuring* clients is not in the spirit of being client-centred, for reassurance does not respect client autonomy and self-direction, is judgemental, and often involves a frame of reference external to the client.

Secondly, and on a quite different level, consider the situation where a therapist reassures a client that 'it will be okay' or 'you are not alone', for instance. Suppose that it will *not* be okay and that despite the therapist's assurances the client still *does* feel alone? The therapist in this example could hardly be said to be respecting the client's world of experiencing and perceptions.

As with so many of these skills and techniques, there would appear to be an anxiety that *not* to use them would result in the therapist being perceived as heartless. *It is really very important to understand and live the difference between an outcome being predictable and striving to achieve that outcome.* If a therapist strives to empathise with and understand a client's world of feelings and meanings, a predictable outcome is that the client will experience being someone worthy of being understood – and the client may well feel reassured by this. However, it is *not* the therapist's *intent* to reassure the client, nor are client feelings of reassurance a goal of client-centred therapy. As Rogers said, if the therapist can *be* the core conditions, the client can *do* the rest.

Probing and questioning

Probing

At one extreme, it is not difficult to see that client-centred therapy has nothing to do with the therapist taking a crowbar to the client in order to jemmy out their feelings or meanings – client-centred therapy is about prizing, not prising! However, clients reflecting upon the process of their therapy often describe it as having been 'like peeling back the layers of onion' until they discovered the 'core' of their personality or being. What part does the counsellor play in this process? After all, the core conditions for client-centred therapy do indicate that the therapist needs, necessarily, to be genuinely interested in (and respectful of) the client's world of feelings and personal meanings. Might *taking a genuine interest* in someone relate to probing in an effort to understand?

Returning to the theme of therapist *intent* might be helpful here. It is true that if the therapist communicates, with some degree of accuracy, authentic and respectful empathic understanding, then the client is likely to respond by taking further steps on their journey of self-discovery. However, the *intent* of the therapist is to strive to sensitively empathise, *not* to somehow 'move a client on'. In other words, a *predictable consequence* of the client perceiving authentic unconditional positive regard and empathic understanding from the therapist is that the client will continue on their journey, going deeper and further if they choose to do so. This is the *if–then* quality of client-centred therapy that was described in Chapter 1 – *if* the client receives nurturing conditions, *then* the client may grow. Just as the phrase '*Why be the magician when you can be the magic?*' emerged:

Why be the gardener when you can be the garden?

Carl Rogers wrote of the 'soil of the theory' out of which client-centred therapy grew. Similarly, maybe the counsellor can provide the soil out of which clients may grow. It might be that counsellor *supervisors* can in part tend the garden, and it might be that therapist personal and professional development activities are important in the process of striving to ensure that conditions in the garden are all that they can be. However, the therapy garden is all that is necessary for the plant to grow – there is no need to prise open or go poking around, whether clumsily or smoothly, in the petals.

Questioning

> During one post-workshop discussion, a participant said to Rogers, 'I noticed that you asked questions of the client. But just last night a lecturer told us we must never do that'. Rogers responded, 'Well, I'm in the fortunate position of not having to be a Rogerian'.
>
> (Brink, personal communication, 1990,
> quoted in Farber *et al.* 1996: p. 11)

Carl Rogers and his colleagues discovered through their research activities that a distinguishing feature of client-centred counselling was that the therapist frames far fewer communications as questions than is the case with most (if not all) other approaches to psychotherapy. Likewise, at the commencement of client-centred therapy training courses (or at the end of counselling skills programmes), it is not uncommon for something in excess of 90% of trainee counsellor communications to their clients to be phrased as questions. On skills courses that purport to be 'client-centred' (or 'person-centred' or 'humanistic' or 'non-directive') most of these questions will be open-ended – yet a *question*, whether 'open' or 'open-ended' or otherwise, *cannot and does not convey empathy or understanding*.

If, for instance, therapists have empathically understood clients, why would they then need to question them? Just how respectful of client feelings and meanings is it when, after a client has just described the most harrowing and dreadful experiences, the therapist says 'How do you feel about that?'. Furthermore, there are repercussions to asking questions in *process* terms, for *if* the counsellor asks questions, the onus is *then* upon the client to reply to those questions – in other words, the *counsellor* is leading the session, not the *client*. As a consequence of this therapist question–client answer–therapist question–client answer pattern, the client could be forgiven for inferring that if all of the therapist's questions are adequately answered, a solution will be given to the client by the therapist, or if not a solution, at least an accurate prognosis or diagnosis, or whatever. Yet another consequence is that if the therapist's capacities are, to whatever extent, engaged with formulating their next question to the client, how fully is the client being heard? How fully is the therapist striving to respect, empathise and understand?

To illustrate this point, many trainee therapists have, over the years, commented that when they were tape recording counselling practice sessions, they felt a need to 'perform' and to 'get it right', and they usually believed that the tape-recorded evidence was not accurately reflecting their usual practice. In other words, their capacities were largely devoted to *formulating responses*, rather than really listening, really hearing and really striving to respectfully enter their clients' worlds of feelings and meanings. However, by the end of successful client-centred therapy training, *less than 5%* of therapist communications are questions. Instead, the therapist *communicates* (albeit it tentatively and cautiously at times) empathic understanding rather than *responding* to clients with open-ended questions, or reflections, or by paraphrasing or summarising what the client has just said.

Please note that this is not to say that the client-centred therapist *never* asks questions. A general guideline is that a client-centred way of being is only to ask a question when no empathy is being experienced, and the question asked is designed to *generate* empathic understanding. This guideline can be refined somewhat, too, for Carl Rogers wrote about empathic *guessing* and empathic *inference*. That is, it is not as simple as an instant 'no empathy – therefore ask' – there is no 'if–then' formula here (as in *if* there is no empathy being experienced, *then* ask a question in order to gain some). Rather it is a case of striving to gather and absorb *all* client cues (verbal, paraverbal and non-verbal) in an attempt to enter their frame of reference. A tentative guess or inference is preferable to a non-empathic question (no matter how open-ended).

Therapist self-disclosure

'Letting it all hang out?'

It is true to say that during the course of his career Carl Rogers did change his views somewhat with regard to the therapist's *presence*. In the early days, Carl wrote on many occasions of the need for therapists to 'set their selves aside' when with clients, as typified when he quoted Nat Raskin:

> the counselor makes a maximum effort to get under the skin of the person with whom he is communicating, he tries to get *within* and to live the attitudes expressed instead of observing them, to catch every nuance of their changing nature; in a word, to absorb himself completely in the attitudes of the other. And in struggling to do this, there is simply no room for any other type of counsellor activity or attitude.
> (Raskin, quoted in Rogers 1951: p. 29)

In 1951, Rogers himself wrote:

> the relationship is experienced as a one-way affair in a very unique sense. The whole relationship is composed of the self of the client, the counselor being depersonalized for the purposes of therapy into being 'the client's other self'. It is this warm willingness on the part of the counselor to lay his own self temporarily aside, in order to enter into the experience of the client, which makes the relationship a com-

pletely unique one, unlike anything in the client's previous experience.

(Rogers 1951: p. 208)

However, within just a few years Rogers came to realise that the quality of therapist presence was a very significant factor in counselling, and by the end of his career he was speaking with Gay Barfield of *reciprocal* empathy (as we saw in Chapter 1) rather than 'a one-way affair', and in 1985 he was able to say:

> I think congruence means that one is aware of what one is experiencing inside, and consequently one is able to express it if it seems appropriate in the situation. The most important part is that one is aware of what one is experiencing. And experiencing, as we have said, has both content and feeling in it.
>
> (Rogers and Teich 1992: p. 62)

We might again refer to John Shlien's phrase 'fatuous alternatives in the name of congruence' when looking at appropriate and inappropriate therapist self-disclosure within a client-centred framework, for regrettably there are those who seem to view 'being appropriately congruent' as meaning that it is perfectly in order (or 'appropriate') for the client-centred therapist to 'let it all hang out' (a kind of 'anything goes' approach to therapy). Such people, it seems, can try to justify just about *anything* by saying 'I was just *being* congruent' or, worse still, 'I was just *communicating* my congruence'! Well, maybe it is true that such a person *is being* congruent, yet it is also true to say that this congruence hardly deeply encapsulates unconditional positive regard and empathic understanding. As Rogers stated:

> For therapy to occur the wholeness of the therapist in the relationship is primary, but a part of the congruence of the therapist must be the experience of unconditional positive regard and the experience of empathic understanding.
>
> (Rogers 1959: p. 215)

'I was just communicating my congruence' is worse still because it demonstrates a complete lack of understanding about what congruence in a client-centred framework *means* and *is*. Carl Rogers maintained that much of our experiencing is *available* to awareness (given the right conditions – more of this in Chapter 4), and congruence is a lack of *denying* significant experiencing to awareness, or not having to *distort* our experiencing in order to allow it into our awareness. To 'communicate congruence' to a client, a therapist would need to be saying something like 'Right now, I am denying none of my significant experiencing to my awareness, nor am I distorting it in order to permit it into my awareness, albeit in a skewed fashion' – this is not very likely or appropriate, nor is it very *client*-centred! Nor was therapist communication or client perception of therapist congruence initially one of the six conditions for therapeutic personality change. It was only deemed necessary for the client to receive the therapist's unconditional positive regard and empathic understanding (the fourth and fifth conditions), because at the time Rogers was less certain about the place of therapist disclosure. The notion of therapist congruence will be more fully explored later, but for now let it be stated that *there is a crucial difference between communicating congruence* and *congruent communication*. Thus while disclosing that there is no denial or distortion of significant experiencing of the therapist by the therapist is both highly unlikely and undesirable, it *is* highly desirable that the client experiences the therapist's respect and empathy as *authentic* because it *is* authentic – that is, congruent.

When speaking of the personal growth journey that is an ingredient (and probably the main ingredient) on the way to becoming client-centred, Carl did say that it was regrettable that some people never moved beyond the *self–self–self* phase (Berwick and Rogers 1983). Some members of the Center for Studies of the Person came up with the idea of a 'narcissistic paradigm' (*this is what I want, so to hell with you!*). Perhaps a 'masochistic paradigm' is worthy of mention, too (*this is what you want, so to hell with me!*). Quite frequently, internalised conditions of worth about pleasing others lead to the thwarting of the actualising tendency – the person lives their life as a server, a carer, a tender of others, hence the *masochistic paradigm* (what I want, need or desire is of meagre merit compared with catering to the needs of others). One of the predictable process phases in client-centred therapy is a movement *away from* values introjected from others, a movement away from pleasing others and *towards* pleasing the self, hence the *narcissistic paradigm* (my wants, needs or desires clearly take precedence over those of others). It is crucial to realise that *this phase does not constitute the entire journey,* and, as Rogers conceded, there are those who emerge from training and other person-centred experiences not having moved beyond *self–self–self.* Just as it is conceivable that the learning of counselling skills *might* represent steps along the way towards becoming empathic as a way of being, so entering a narcissistic phase might be a process movement towards (client-centred) congruence. Nevertheless, let us be clear that the counsellor 'letting it all hang out' or believing that 'anything goes' is not what Rogers meant client-centred therapy to be. Such attitudes are more akin to Shlien's 'fatuous alternatives'.

However, this is not to say that the client-centred therapist is a 'closed book' or a 'blank screen'. As already stated, it has been extremely unfortunate that some people seem to take words like 'transparency' and 'genuineness' or phrases like 'being real' to also mean 'let it all hang out' or 'anything goes'. *Being transparently real is only client-centred if the therapist has deeply integrated the core conditions as a way of therapeutic being.* This is not the same as stating that the client-centred therapist *never* self-discloses. When asked by John Masterson about the danger of personal growth journeys resulting in everything else having to stop this instant (perhaps 'a fatuous alternative in the name of immediacy') until personal feelings are worked through, Rogers said:

> I've seen that happen, yes. . . . The risk runs two ways. Sometimes what people learn is to be more expressive of their feelings – period. Sometimes what they learn is to be more willing to listen, and to hear – and then perhaps sit on their own feelings. Either is a risk and unfortunate. I think it has to be a balance: of being willing to express what I deeply feel, but also a willingness to hear what you deeply feel – and that I think is the basis for a stronger, richer relationship, when there is that balance.
>
> (Rogers 1985)

Appropriate therapist self-disclosure

Carl Rogers gave us useful guidelines on when it might be appropriate for a therapist to self-disclose, the primary reason being when *not* to do so would serve to block the therapist's capacity to absorb, empathise and understand – when the therapist is prevented from meaningfully entering a client's world of feelings or meanings due to some personal experiencing acting as a barrier across the gateway to the experiencing and meanings of another. However, Rogers also believed that if a therapist feeling is experienced as *persistent* and *prolonged* in the relationship, then it probably merits being voiced *in* that relationship. He quoted the experience of a colleague who, near the end of his working day, received a call saying that his son had sustained minor injuries in a road traffic accident. With only one client to see, and knowing that his son was in no dire danger, the therapist believed that he could set aside his own feelings and thoughts until later. However, during the therapy session the counsellor's feelings and thoughts *did* veer towards his injured child so, after some internal mulling over, he thought it best to 'come clean' with the client – who responded by expressing relief, because they had perceived the therapist's distraction as meaning that it was something 'unattractive' about them that had elicited a negative reaction from the therapist.

To *refrain* from self-disclosure might be anti-therapeutic:

> From the beginning, and with increasing emphasis as time has passed, Rogers has stressed the centrality of sincerity, honesty, and genuineness in the therapist's responses. It is only his genuinely felt understanding and honest positive regard that can be deeply helpful and curative; technique alone is not enough and may even be irrelevant or harmful at certain moments in psychotherapy. If, for instance, the therapist uses his nondirectiveness as a way of suppressing his own annoyance because the poor weak client couldn't possibly take it, an attitude of fundamental disrespect, annoyance, and lack of real regard for the client's powers will be communicated. Even with the best of intentions, such communication of lack of understanding and regard is damaging because the sneaky obscurity of it tends to poison the atmosphere and inhibit that flow of honest feeling that is at the heart of client-centered help.
>
> (Barton 1974: p. 195)

For a therapist to *feign* empathic understanding (perhaps by reverting to skills and techniques) or to offer only a *semblance* of unconditional positive regard would not be *authentic* self-expression – the therapist is not a whole person, the therapist is *incongruent*. Carl Rogers said that respect for the capacity of individuals was a central tenet that permeated his whole being, so when being a whole person in the counselling relationship:

> I still feel that the person who should guide the client's life is the client. My whole philosophy and whole approach is to try to strengthen him in that way of being, that he's in charge of his own life and nothing that I say is intended to take that capacity or that opportunity away from him. It is changed in this respect, that I would try to be aware of my own feelings and express them as my feelings without imposing

them on him. I would express even negative feelings. I might tell a client, 'I'm really bored by what you're saying'. It doesn't guide him. It does provide him with some rather jolting data which he must handle in some way or another. But I'm not telling him what he should do to avoid boring me. Maybe he would just as soon bore me; that's up to him . . . I was quite fascinated by the discovery that people did have much more capacity to guide themselves than I'd given them credit for. I became sort of a tourist in that, thinking 'Let's not let any of me into the situation except just an understanding of the client's feelings'. I gradually realized over the years that the tourist approach shakes the client out of what might be a very close interpersonal relationship which is much more rewarding.

(Rogers and Evans 1975: pp. 26–7)

Rogers also wrote of experiencing yet being unaware of annoyance:

When I am experiencing an attitude of annoyance toward another person but am unaware of it, then my communication contains contradictory messages. My words are giving one message, but I am also in subtle ways communicating the annoyance I feel, and this confuses the other person and makes him distrustful, though he too may be unaware of what is causing the difficulty. When . . . I fail to listen to what is going on in me, fail because of my own defensiveness to sense my own feelings, then this kind of failure seems to result. It has made it seem to me that the most basic learning for anyone who hopes to establish any kind of helping relationship is that it is safe to be transparently real.

(Rogers 1961: p. 51)

Rogers followed this by writing that, strange as it may seem, it is helpful if a therapist can be his or her own therapist. We shall see that one outcome of therapy is that clients become more self-accepting, and an outcome of that outcome is that they become more accepting towards others. The person who has achieved unconditional positive self-regard in a responsible and socialised way through a process of being sensitively aware of, respectful of and under-standing towards their own inner feelings has moved significantly towards being the necessary and sufficient conditions for being a client-centred therapist. Rogers continued:

Now, acceptantly to be what I am, in this sense, and to permit this to show through to the other person, is the most difficult task I know and one I never fully achieve. But to realize that this *is* my task has been most rewarding because it has helped me to find what has gone wrong with interpersonal relationships which have become snarled and to put them on a constructive track again. It has meant that if I am to facilitate the personal growth of others in relation to me, then I must grow, and while this is often painful, it is also enriching.

(Rogers 1961: p. 51)

In other words, if a feeling (or attitude) is persistent enough or strong enough in a relationship, it will probably be sensed by clients anyway (this could be viewed as an example of the 'reciprocal empathy' referred to in Chapter 1), so honesty and openness are preferable to the alarm or insecurity that the therapist being a 'closed book' might generate. However, such honesty springs from the integrity of the therapist, and that integrity includes the deep embodiment of a client-centred way of being.

Let us close this section with three final quotes about Carl Rogers that hopefully capture the essence of congruent therapist communication. The first illustrates his total commitment to entering and being with clients in their own personal worlds of experiencing:

> It is interesting to note that, after a demonstration interview, Rogers would occasionally tell his audience that his attention was so totally focussed on his client that the rest of the world simply disappeared for him.
>
> (Brink, cited in Farber *et al.* 1996: p. 30)

Next comes a quote that resonates with my own experience and with comments made by several associates. In it we can see how self-disclosures made by Rogers were very much located in and relevant to the client's world of feelings and meanings:

> One of our recorded clients in our research said at the last interview 'I really don't know you at all, and I've never known anyone better in my life'. And both things could be true. She didn't know anything about me as a person outside of therapy, but in therapy she knew me as someone who was understanding and real.
>
> (Rogers and Russell 2002: p. 286)

Finally, Rogers spoke of his regret at not emphasising the rigorous and disciplined nature of being client-centred:

> Being real does not involve us doing anything we want to do; it means a disciplined approach. That's one thing that I realize I have not stressed enough, and consequently it has been overlooked. I'm quite a disciplined person myself, and it comes naturally to me to think that everyone else is, too, but that's not so.
>
> (Rogers and Russell 2002: p. 286)

Transference and counter-transference

The view of Carl Rogers with regard to the theories of transference and counter-transference was unequivocally clear – they were unfounded and had outlived their time. Carl deplored them, believing them to be seductively disgusting and socially reprehensible. *There is no place at all for such thinking or practice in client-centred therapy.*

> I have a very strong conviction that psychoanalysis is a speculative, outdated theory which still hangs on, which has an incredible amount of undue importance in the training of psychiatrists and social workers. I think it is absurd that it hasn't been displaced.
>
> (Rogers and Russell 2002: p. 243)

If psychoanalysis, including such theories of 'transference' and 'counter-transference' (and 'resistance', too) are so repugnant, why are they still with us? Carl's opinion with regard to their continuing influence was as follows:

> I think it is because it appeals to a certain type of mind. Some people feel something simple must obviously be untrue or low grade, but if you have a complicated theory that nobody can quite understand, and it's really mysterious, and it takes an expert to even spell it out, and the way it applies to an individual is so complicated that it would take years and years to really understand it – 'Ah, that must be true'.
>
> (Rogers and Russell 2002: p. 243)

While some people might think that it 'must be true' because it is complex and long-winded in its learning, Carl Rogers believed there to be a distinct lack of meaningful research data to back up the alleged importance of so-called transference in therapy, and indeed a reluctance on the part of practitioners for whom 'transference' is a fundamental aspect of their counselling to open their data to public scrutiny. Carl's opinion was that:

> To deal with transference feelings as a very special part of therapy, making their handling the very core of therapy, is to my mind a grave mistake. Such an approach fosters dependency and lengthens therapy. It creates a whole new problem, the only purpose of which appears to be the intellectual satisfaction of the therapist – showing the elaborateness of his or her expertise. I deplore it.
>
> (Rogers 1987b: p. 183)

Looking at notions of 'transference' and 'counter-transference', Carl differentiated between two main types of client feelings or emotions towards the therapist, namely *feelings that are an understandable client response to the attitudes and behaviours of the therapist*, and *feelings that have little or no relationship with or to the therapist*. Thus a client might understandably feel anger or resentment at the therapist offering (premature) interpretations, or projecting an aura of expertness or superiority, or a client might understandably feel warmth or love when experiencing a deep understanding from the counsellor. Such feelings are *understandable* client responses to a client-centred therapeutic relationship. On the other hand, feelings such as love, sexual desire, adoration, hatred, contempt, fear and mistrust are projections *from* the client, they may be positive or negative, and they are usually 'transferred' from a 'significant other', or indeed they may be aspects of the client's self that the client cannot as yet accept. Furthermore, in psychoanalysis, client attitudes that are 'transferred' to the current therapeutic relationship are usually deemed to be infantile in nature and origin, and hence link with Freudian theories about psychosexual development – theories that play no part whatsoever in the client-centred framework.

In addition, Carl also stated that even if the phenomena described as transference and counter-transference become discernible, 'In client-centered therapy, however, this involved and persistent dependent transference relationship does not tend to develop' (Rogers 1951: p. 201), indicating that so-called transference phenomena might be more to do with the practitioner and the relationships that practitioners create than with some 'universal fact' of human relations. Carl proposed that *it is not necessary* for the therapist to determine whether client feelings and emotions are counsellor-caused or projections, stating that while such deliberations may be of theoretical interest, they are not problematic in client-centred therapy theoretically, for:

> A true transference relationship is perhaps most likely to occur when the client experiences another as having a more effective understanding of his own self than he himself possesses.
>
> (Rogers 1951: p. 218)

Carl also stated that there was *absolutely no need* to make 'transferred' attitudes 'special', or to permit the dependence that features so prominently in other (especially psychoanalytic) approaches. Instead, the client-centred therapist can *accept* dependent feelings, thereby not colluding with client attempts to change the counsellor's role. In other words, accurate understanding and genuine acceptance, together with non-evaluation, non-judging and non-interpretation, result in a tendency for 'transference' attitudes to dissolve, with the feelings becoming expressed towards their true object, thus resulting in greater client awareness of and new insights into the meanings of experience.

Linking a belief in and a therapeutic focus on so-called transference with the psychoanalytic notion of 'resistance', Carl also differentiated between an *understandable* resistance to the often painful process of admitting to awareness previously denied and distorted experience (as happens in client-centred therapy), and resistance *to* the therapist created *by* the therapist (as occurs in more Freudian-based therapies). Transference and resistance are interpreted *by* the therapist, usually serving no really useful purpose other than to satisfy the intellectual curiosity of the therapist (and maybe make the therapist appear very clever). Focusing on such phenomena as 'transference' and 'counter-transference' (if they even exist), interpreting them and dealing with the resistance created by the therapist's interpretations, therapeutically seems to have one main function – to needlessly prolong the counselling.

Why then might notions of so-called transference and counter-transference seem to keep re-emerging as somehow desirable, even among so-called client-centred practitioners? Why is it that every so often we hear yet another speaker, or read yet another article, which suggests that transference and counter-transference could be incorporated into client-centred therapy with no loss of integrity? Could it be that Carl was right when he said that maybe some therapists *do* experience a need to be perceived as exceptionally clever and smart by either their clients or their peers, as knowing far more about client psychological processes and experiencing than clients themselves can possibly know or discover? Might there be something in the links made by Carl Rogers and Gay Barfield to the problem-solving, mechanically and technologically orientated nature of the so-called 'developed countries'? Perhaps we can let Carl have the last word on transference:

> I feel there's something about its complexity that is very seductive and disgusting. I get really upset – perhaps that word should not be used. But it is socially reprehensible that the professions have not moved beyond psychoanalysis.
>
> (Rogers and Russell 2002: p. 244)

Rogers passionately believed that the 'special virtue' of client-centred therapy is that *the client has no need to resist the therapist*, as the *client* is free to deal with any resistances found within the self.

Uh-huh

One of the more gross caricatures of client-centred therapy is that the therapist has a bouncy rubber spring for a neck, and simply sits there nodding and bobbing sagely, interjecting the occasional (but well-timed) 'hm-mm' and 'uh-huh'! It gets worse – despite all that we have learned from Carl Rogers about *thou shalt not skill*, and how *non*-client-centred it is to direct or manipulate clients, many counselling skills and, regrettably, counsellor training courses teach students 'minimal encouragers' or therapist *noises* as *techniques* designed to *encourage* the client to talk.

It may well be that if you are listening to someone very attentively, closely tracking their every word, gesture and movement, and striving to sense, absorb and understand the feelings and personal meanings that 'lie behind' client words from within their frame of reference, then you may well utter the odd 'mm' or 'uh-huh' or whatever noise comes naturally for you, but what a far cry this is from using noises like 'uh-huh' and 'hm-mm' as *techniques designed to get the client to do something!*

Here is another minimal noise:

Sigh . . .

Understanding about

It may seem somewhat surprising that *understanding* is included in a 'The client-centred counsellor does not' section of a book on empathic understanding! Carl Rogers believed that therapist communications from an external frame of reference were not necessarily 'wrong', 'bad' or to be decried, stressing that such communications are usually sympathetic – coming, as it were, from a good, understandable place. Indeed, he wrote that often such sympathetic communications are:

> even attempts to 'understand', in the sense of 'understanding about', rather than 'understanding with'. The locus of perceiving is, however, outside of the client.
>
> (Rogers 1951: p. 33)

Understanding about is perhaps best characterised by the '*You (feel) – because – (reason)*' exercise that is sometimes employed in counselling *skills* training. For instance, the person utilising this skill might say something like 'You *feel* angry *because* it seems so unfair'. The learning of such techniques may or may not represent a step on the way towards becoming empathic (perhaps for some trainees it does and for others it does not). However, this type of *response* demonstrates that the helper understands *why it is that the other person feels the way that they do*. It does *not* communicate that the listener has absorbed what the sensations of anger feel like to the client, or what personal meanings lie behind the notion of justice for that client. For instance, 'You *feel* sad *because* your partner has just died' states the obvious – it does not communicate an *as if* feeling of grief or a sensitive understanding of what this *means* to the client. With client-centred empathy:

> the client himself has been the source of understanding; he, *from his own point of view*, can gradually articulate the sense and meaning of his difficulties. Hence, there is no need for an elaborate developmental theory or complex theory of neurosis for an effective understanding of the client. The client can be helped to explain himself, to give an account of his own world, and it is *his* account, *his* description, *his* developing consciousness, and *his* expression of feeling that will make most ample sense of his life.
>
> (Barton 1974: p. 179)

Moving beyond *understanding about* and towards an *empathic way of being* is essential for the client-centred therapist.

Quack of all trades, master of none?

If we are to be *client*-centred, perhaps it might be as well to listen to our *clients*. In personal correspondence (later made public), Professor Dave Mearns wrote:

> I am concerned and frustrated at the bad name which is attaching to person-centred practice in Britain. An example is the fact that complaints against 'person-centred' members of BAC [the British Association for Counselling] far outweigh those of any other discipline, even taking into account the fact that more people ascribe to the person-centred approach than any other core model. Particularly frustrating is the fact that when you scratch beneath the surface of these complaints you almost always find that the practitioner has virtually no training in the approach . . .
>
> (Dave Mearns, quoted in Vincent 1998: p. 1)

In the UK at least, there has been a major increase in counsellor training programmes that describe themselves as 'eclectic' or 'humanistic' or, most commonly, as 'integrative'. The vast majority of them aim at just above the minimum hours requirement for validation or accreditation. So in what usually amounts to a course of around 450 hours in total, it is maintained that trainees can come to grips with, thoroughly understand and competently practise two or often three 'mainstream' approaches to therapy – that's either 225 hours or 150 hours per approach. *Why?* Why, oh why, oh why?

Do trainers who offer such programmes genuinely, honestly and deeply believe that the best interests of clients are served by 150 to 225 hours of training in each approach? Do trainers maintain this belief (and their integrity) even in the light of research evidence which demonstrates that 'hotchpotch' counsellors (many of whom call themselves 'person-centred' because it seems to be the most embracing label) attract a disproportionate number of client complaints? Or might this be down to market forces ('buy two, get one free' and 'it's more attractive to punters if they think they're getting more')? Might this even be due to there being some trainers who enjoy 'strutting their stuff', and the more stuff there is to strut the better? Whatever the reason or reasons, it is clearly bad news both for clients and for authentic client-centred therapists.

Some further evidence can be cited. A local counselling directory (Hampshire Association for Counselling 2001) contains the details of 91 counsellors, of whom just under one-third offer therapy rooted in a single approach, and of these, three counsellors are identified as client-centred and three as person-centred. The average number of approaches offered by the rest of the counsellors is slightly over three. Around 30% of the counsellors offered two different approaches, over 15% offered three different approaches, 18% offered four different approaches, and 4% offered five different approaches. Over 40% of these 'eclectic' counsellors included 'client-centred', 'person-centred' or 'Rogerian' (a term Rogers disliked) in their descriptions. Yet Carl Rogers believed that the use of different techniques and styles with the same or with different therapeutic styles actually destroys the potential for a truly therapeutic relationship with clients (Rogers and Sanford 1985), so how with any integrity can *client-centred* or *person-centred* be included in the description of an 'integrative' counsellor? We know, too, that Rogers gave us necessary *and sufficient* conditions to work within.

Carl identified two further drawbacks, the first being the trainee counsellor who becomes 'mesmerised' by or idolises a trainer, therapist or even an approach to counselling. Such people, said Carl, tend not to think for and *be* themselves:

> The other – and this is an equal danger, I feel – is when people say 'Well, I'm an eclectic therapist; I do whatever seems necessary'. That tends to mean they have no theoretical basis by which they're operating, so they have no way of determining whether they're really doing the right things or not. They sort of fly by the seat of their pants, which has certain good qualities, but also very grave deficiencies . . . The need is to think about theory, expand theory, expand hypotheses, but to do it in a thoughtful and coherent way.
>
> (Rogers and Russell 2002: p. 275)

It seems, then, that there are external threats to the integrity of client-centred therapy – for instance, from people who 'use' the core conditions some of the time or with some of their clients, or who see being client-centred as a 'good basis for the relationship' but not *sufficient* to resolve all client concerns. Sadly, there are threats from within, too. We have already looked at issues surrounding those who seem to think that being congruent means 'anything goes', or who claim to use client-centred 'reflecting' skills. When Carl Rogers was asked about 'using anything and everything', he said:

> I think that in many ways it can and, in some respects, has gone completely wild, and I regret that. In its more solid aspects, it's one of the most significant social inventions of this century because it is a way of eliminating alienation and loneliness, of getting people into better communication with one another, of helping them develop fresh insights into themselves, and helping them get feedback from others so that they perceive how they are received by others. It serves a great many useful purposes.
>
> (Rogers and Evans 1975: p. 32)

Rogers went on to say that the reputation of the person-centred approach (he was talking at the time about broader applications, not just therapy) could be damaged in the public eye.

It may well be that our reputations *have* been damaged and *continue* to be damaged by these internal and external threats to client-centred integrity. However, we can live by our own beliefs – rather than be defensive, let us celebrate what and who and how we are.

> Anyway, I think that because I'm not trying to do all these fancy things that other therapists do, I have a more complete freedom to really enter the world of the client.
>
> (Rogers and Russell 2002: p. 281)

Summary

The importance of not seeing counselling or therapy as a skills-based activity is clear from the fact that when, near the end of his life, Carl Rogers was asked whether he had any regrets, he replied:

> I regret that in early writings about therapy we were so fascinated with the enormous learnings from recording interviews that we became too much focussed on techniques, and that has misled a great many people in the counseling field. I realize that.
>
> (Rogers 1989: p. 198)

Furthermore, to take a principled stance *against* skills and techniques places the therapist in a minority, for:

> Contrary to the opinion of a great many psychotherapists, I have long held that it is not the technical skill or training of the therapist that determines his success. Instead, I believe it is the presence of certain attitudes in the therapist, which are communicated to, and perceived by, his client, that effect success in psychotherapy.
>
> (Rogers 1989: p. 10)

There is clearly an essential difference between *being skilled* and the *implementation of skills*. Being skilled is something that someone *is*, whereas implementing skills is something that someone *does* to another person. Witness Carl Rogers in action and you will most likely experience someone who is extremely skilled not only at *being* authentically respectful and understanding, but also at *communicating* genuine acceptance and empathy. The therapist who has *got* (or acquired) the skills and techniques to *use* on or apply to clients tends to *respond* by utilising tools that are designed to *do* or achieve some desired result.

There is an anecdote about an audience watching Rogers demonstrate client-centred therapy. One viewer turns to another and says 'Boy! That Carl Rogers! He sure has got it!'. After a reflective pause comes the reply 'No . . . He hasn't *got* it – he *is* it'.

Chapter 3

Empathising in action: an inter-view

Background to this inter-view

During a diploma group, a counsellor trainee asked me to describe, 'off the cuff' so to speak, my *process* of empathising. The questioner spoke of having learned all about definitions, academic understanding and the theory of empathy (such as the place of empathic understanding within client-centred therapeutic process), and had experienced both the giving and receiving of empathy in personal therapy, in practice sessions and on a client work placement. Yet this trainee was really curious about *what actually happens within a therapist when that therapist is engaged in empathising.* Although I recall feeling somewhat 'put on the spot', there was also a simultaneous experiencing of curiosity as my mind engaged with the quality of the question, followed by the thought that it deserved a full and honest answer. So . . . I took a deep breath and spoke. A dynamic dialogue ensued, in which questioners were encouraged to reflect upon their own experiencing, with further questions being put by group members, which in turn triggered further exploration, clarification and ideas.

A couple of days later I started trying to remember and type up what I had said. I recall feeling somewhat abashed in that I was quite interested in my own answers! What had emerged from the dialogue felt useful – a pulling together of some of the strands of 'empathising in action', if you will. As the session felt a bit like an interview at the time, I thought 'Who can I get to interview me?'. As I started typing, I framed the first sentence as the initial question that had been asked in the training group. Then I thought 'Why not interview myself?'. This idea seemed a little crazy at first, but I nevertheless persevered, and the process turned out to feel quite dynamic. A college manager reminded me, when I happened to mention my feeling of silliness, of 'FAQs' ('Frequently Asked Questions') computerised systems, and I became more aware that it might actually be helpful to remember and collate questions about empathic understanding that trainees have posed over the years, and to attempt to respond to them fully and honestly.

So what follows is in part an interview with Steve Vincent, in which he responds to questions put to him by . . . Steve Vincent! Many of the questions are ones I recollect trainees and other peers having asked over the years; some of the questions are my own. This process of exploring *what actually happens within the therapist when empathising* has since been repeated in other groups and in further dialogues, and some of these sessions were tape recorded and transcribed. Here, then, is an edited version of responses to questions about empathy in action – an interview drawn from a variety of sources. I hope that it has meaning and relevance.

Empathy: an inter-view

I Would you be prepared to describe for us your process of empathising?

Well . . . I realise that I might sound a little like a stereotyped politician, but first of all I'd like to amend the question somewhat! I think that it makes more sense for me to try and describe my process of *striving* to empathise . . . Yes, this has more meaning, for it seems to me that what is most therapeutic is an *authentic striving* to empathise, rather than some kind of 'effortless and accurate' empathy *all of the time*. If we think in terms of being a compassionate companion to the client, for example, I will be journeying *alongside* rather than knowing or showing the way . . . something like that. Maybe there is something, too, about empathy being very hard work, and a place we strive to reach rather than a place we instantly find ourselves at. Maybe the journey to get there is as important as the arrival.

Anyway, I'm with a client. I think one of the primary and . . . No, let me step back a minute . . . I'm *not* with a client. Maybe there is something about preparing myself *before* I meet with the client in person. I am reminded of some of the clinical psychology research into receptiveness. In one experiment a volunteer group was divided into two equal halves, one half being told that pain would be administered at a set time, the other half being kept in the dark. When the pain was administered, those who had received prior warning experienced the pain more keenly – both subjectively and physiologically (through scientific measurement) – so the discovery was that our brains can be 'primed' to be ready to receive stimuli and sensations. So maybe something similar could be true for empathising. Maybe if I prepare myself to receive then I will perceive more keenly. This is one reason why I am all in favour of the 50-minute counselling hour! I use the space between meeting with clients to calm myself in different ways – mentally and physically. I remember now, I think Professor Susan Greenfield called this 'mental priming process' *modulation* (Greenfield 2000). For me, regrettably, this often means slipping out of the back for a cigarette and a pace around, and during that time I usually kind of mentally freewheel. It feels, when I look back at it, rather as if I am emptying myself of the last client (maybe a kind of storing, rather than a forgetting) in order to be as open as I can be to receiving the next one. I do experience myself after this short break as somehow freshened up and ready to meet with whatever comes through the door next. So I'm not smoking, I'm modulating!

Not only is there something about my own experience, but also it would not surprise me in the least if this kind of receptivity is physiologically or neurologically (or whatever) measurable. There may well be reliable clinical back-up research data to support the view that 'priming' could be a significant factor in preparing to *empathise*. It occurs to me that this view could be backed up by looking at its opposite, too. Just a few days ago I joined a group an hour or so after it had started. Although my late arrival was expected (it had been negotiated and agreed well in advance), I nevertheless felt relatively disconnected from the group for quite some time. It occurs to me, too, that I simply drove up, parked, and rushed in. As I speak, I feel sure that other factors were also relevant here (factors that I shall not go into right now as they do not feel appropriate), yet it seems to me that part of my feeling of disconnection was due to my not being adequately primed. I think that I tend to trust my experience in this – I sense that there is something very real and true in the significance of modulating my mind to receive empathically.

So where was I? Now I *am* primed and meet with a client. I think one of the primary and initial inner processes is that I am uncluttered and receptive, and that enables me to strive to *absorb* all that is passing between us, and primarily all that a client is communicating. I will strive to be watchful, in that I think it really helps to look at the person who is communicating! I strive to be attentive to the eyes, the mouth, the face, the head, the body, the hands and arms, the feet . . . And this is not some 'detached observing' that takes place. Rather I am trying to absorb all that the client is experiencing from moment to moment. I recall watching a Carl Rogers demonstration session, in which he began a communication with 'I gather . . .', and I liked that – the therapist strives to *gather* all that a client is giving off and giving out. Gathering includes absorbing *sounds* as well as vision and words. For instance, how is a client speaking? What is the quality of a client's silence? There is a *whole universe* of communication to absorb . . .

2 Can you clarify some of this by giving an example now?

Of what? I'm sorry, I see that some of you are looking quizzical or puzzled. Yet there are so many aspects to this universe of communication! I shall try to bring in examples as we go along.

Okay, I recall a demonstration session last year where I was one of a couple being counselled. The therapist missed the 'discreet' tears of my partner. Those tears were communicating something and the therapist was unaware of that communication, let alone what the crying might feel like or what personal meanings might underlie this weeping. Come to think of it, the therapist totally missed what it felt like or what it meant to me, too! I recall another instance where a client was saying nothing out loud, but her fingers were kind of trammelling (the movement that a cat's paws and claws often make) the arm of the chair. I not only noticed this, I actually (unobtrusively) made the same movement myself, in an attempt to gain some kind of insight into what she might be experiencing. I think I often *gaze* at clients when we first meet. I certainly don't *stare* in some kind of *piercing* way – I like the idea of a *gentle gaze*. I hope that this gentle gaze conveys that I am interested, curious and wanting to absorb. At least, I hope that some clients sense something of this, if they look! As I think about it, I feel that in initial meetings many clients are too absorbed in what is going on for them to notice very much of my intentions. Maybe as therapy progresses clients sense more of my countenance and what it means. Anyway, my hope is that if clients do look at me, my face (and perhaps especially my eyes) will let them accurately discern *something* of my intentions. (I'm not sure where this comes from, but I remember someone writing about how utterly weird and bizarre it is that two lumps of fatty gristle could communicate so much – yet the eyes do very often seem to say a great deal.)

So I *see* things, I do not just *hear* things. Sometimes what I see might not be what is being voiced. For instance, a client might look ashamed or embarrassed as they are speaking, yet they do not use the words shame or embarrassment. If I am striving to absorb what the client is *experiencing* in the moment, then their embarrassment or shame is as much a part of their being as their words.

3 Doesn't what you have said involve a degree of interpretation? How truly client-centred is that?

I suppose that depends upon your interpretation of interpretation! I guess that there are different degrees of interpretation. It doesn't *feel* like interpretation to me, although it does mean an absorbing and a trying to *sense the sense of* whatever is going on in clients, trying to tune into their sensations and grasp something of what their experiencing means to them. I have come across the phrase 'empathic inference' somewhere, and Rogers wrote of 'empathic guessing' at some point (in 'The Silent Young Man', Chapter 17, Rogers 1967). For me, there is something around . . . If a client *looks*, say, embarrassed, then I think that this is a pretty unequivocal communication. This is not some kind of arrogance about interpretation or some highly intellectualised theory about 'body language', and nor will any communication of empathic inference or guessing be assertive. You don't look convinced . . . okay, let us dwell on this a little longer.

I recall a television programme on the human brain that I saw recently, and one of the statements made was that one of the largest single functions of the brain is given over to face recognition. I don't want to get into pedantic semantics, but I wonder if, at one level at least, there is any kind of subtle difference between *recognition* and *interpretation*. In the Nineteen Propositions (Rogers 1951: pp. 481–533), Carl wrote about internal and external frames of reference, yet he also wrote about a *common frame of reference*, saying that there are *counterparts* of experience in each of us. Many argue that without a common frame of reference, there would be little or no communication at all between us! I am reminded of Maurice Merleau-Ponti, an existentialist philosopher who added *being-within-the-world* to the categories of *being-in-itself* and *being-for-itself*. In other words, there are inanimate objects that have no awareness whatsoever of their own existence (and hence nothing with which to empathise), and there are entities that do have awareness of their own being, yet there is also something about conscious entities (organisms that have awareness of self, others and the world about them) being born into a world where feelings and meanings pre-exist and are absorbed and internalised as we grow into that world within which we share reciprocal relationships. I am also reminded of the idea of the 'I–thou' relationship. There is the 'I', there is the 'thou' and there is a hyphen. Let us not forget the hyphen!

So do I *interpret* a look as meaning 'embarrassed' or do I *recognise* a look as meaning embarrassed? This for me would all seem to link with Carl describing the process of empathising as *perception-checking* – it certainly doesn't feel like a detached observation of client 'body language' coupled with some theoretical belief about what it signifies! And my experience has been that when I have communicated my sensing of client embarrassment to that client – perhaps somewhat tentatively if I feel somewhat uncertain – it is usually accurate or at least *nearly* accurate. And I feel fine with nearly accurate!

4 I'm a little surprised that you have referred to clinical psychology a couple of times already – that doesn't sound like you! Can you say more about that?

It grieves me that so often our focus is so narrow. It grieves me even more that there are those among us who try to develop client-centred therapy by incorporating *old stuff* from other approaches. And by 'old stuff' I mean things like transference, for that seems to rear its ugly head every so often, despite the fact that Rogers *despised* the whole notion of transference!

Yet there is so much that we could be learning and that is compatible with client-centred theory and beliefs! I'm excited, for instance, by the work of Professor Susan Greenfield. Look at Freud. He believed that it was only a matter of time before the physical structures of the id, ego and superego would be found in the human brain. We can say with some certainty that this has turned out to be utter rubbish! Yet what has been discovered, at the 'cutting edge' of neuroscience, if you will, seems to me to bode very well for client-centred therapy – for instance, some of the findings about perception, and how we create the perceptual world around us. Professor Greenfield talks of how nonsensical it is to tie down the development of the self to ages and stages. She writes of what she calls a 'transient self' that is a process of becoming – just like Rogers. I think that it is very important that we pay attention to neuroscientific discoveries and are open to learning from them. I also think that it is *fantastic* that so many of these discoveries are in harmony with client-centred thinking, and that we can develop within our approach without damaging or diluting our integrity.

5 What did you mean by feeling fine with 'nearly accurate' empathy?

Can I step back a moment? It occurs to me that when I said 'You don't look convinced' earlier, that was a live example of what I mean. You didn't *look* convinced, and I voiced my understanding of what your facial expression meant. Subsequent non-verbal signals led me to believe that on this occasion my recognition of your signals was pretty accurate.

Anyway, a few things come to mind about feeling fine with 'nearly accurate' empathy. I am aware of feeling absorbed by the concept of absorbing, so I would like to get back to that before long, too! I remember writing an article called *In Praise Of Being Off-Beam*, the gist of which was that accurate empathy, like a *zap* right between the eyes, is maybe not so therapeutic – or at least persistent and prolonged *zaps* might not be. My experience of offering therapy is of a striving to sensitively enter the world of my client. I venture, sometimes very tentatively, sometimes more confidently, my grasp of what they are experiencing, a grasp that includes, ideally, feelings, thoughts and meanings (and personal meanings may well link with memories). I hope that my empathy and understanding are not *wildly* off-beam, for if my client experiences me as being 'on another planet', then I suspect that the encounter will not be therapeutic for them. So there is something about conditions five and six – that I am actually experiencing a degree of accurate empathic understanding and that the client is receiving this. Therefore constant zaps between the eyes might be inappropriate – too scary, or over-threatening, or whatever. And missing by miles is not too good, either, but if I can get pretty close pretty much of the time – maybe with an occasional *zap* – then that feels good, to me. It's as if the client *knows* that I am striving to sensitively enter their world, and so will be co-operative in that joint venture. If I don't 'get it quite right' then they will clarify for me. And who knows? Maybe in clarifying for me, things will become clearer for them, too.

6 You did a couple of demonstration sessions, and in one I saw you as
   being confident with your empathy, and in the other as really tentative.
   What is that all about?

Well, that's just how it was. I remember the first session well, and I really did feel
reasonably confident that my empathising was fairly accurate, so part of being
authentic was neither to be over-confident nor to be too diffident either. In the
second session I had a heavy cold, and it felt as if I was absorbing through a layer
of cotton wool, so I definitely felt less confident (there was that word 'absorbing'
again! I would like to return to that soon . . .). Yet it occurs to me that even when I
felt more confident I remained kind of . . . humble? That doesn't feel quite right –
maybe a kind of *humility* is incorporated in my way of being, a kind of self-
acceptance that I feel confident about the accuracy of my empathy, yet also
experience a real willingness to be guided by the client. Rogers wrote about
constantly being prepared to change horses in midstream, and Dave Mearns
wrote about the 'dance of psychotherapy'. They both capture some of what I
mean, I think.

Can I just go back to the idea of near enough accurate empathy being good
enough for me for a moment? I am reminded of Carl's adage 'what I am is good
enough', and on one of the CSP/CCTPCAS videos he says more about this. It goes
something like:

> What I am is good enough. And what I am is an imperfect human
> being. Yet imperfect beings can achieve astonishing things. Especially
> when they are aware that they are imperfect beings.
>
> (Rogers and Sanford 1985)

I like that. And it seems to me that the degree of accuracy in my empathic
communications almost feels less important than my striving to be empathic – at
times at least. The outcome may be imperfect, yet if the striving is there, that is
kind of perfect! It's almost as though if I am authentically striving, I can't 'get it
wrong'. If the striving is there, the rest will follow.

You know, it occurs to me that there is also something about *timing* in this
confident or tentative thing. If I reflect on my work with clients, then I think that
it is fair to say that I am less likely to be very tentative the more I have come to get
inside a client's world of feelings and meanings. I will still, I hope, maintain a
degree of humility, but yes – I think that's true. The *less* I know (or the less I have
absorbed or gathered), the more tentative I am likely to be. Of course, if an
ongoing client discloses a completely new aspect, then the tentativeness might
return. So maybe increased confidence and reduced tentativeness is a therapeutic
trend, but not a straight line on a graph, if you see what I mean. Anyway, can I
return to absorbing?

I started off talking about priming myself to be alert, attentive and watchful. I
want to say something more about absorbing *sounds*. By this I mean that I think it
is unfortunate that, over the years, there has perhaps been too much attention
paid to *words*, at the expense of *sounds*. I remember a recent demonstration session
where at one point I voiced something of the client's sense of 'righteous
indignation'. In the audience feedback session that followed, considerable
surprise was expressed because the client had *said nothing* about indignation –

righteous or otherwise – so surely this *couldn't* have been client-centred and *must* have been interpretative or analytic or something. Well, for me the process of 'absorbing' a client includes hearing the *sound* of their communications, and not just the *words* that they speak. When I listened to the *sound* of this client's voice, almost a kind of 'plaintive wailing', the communication of righteous indignation was a strong current that ran through a significant section of the session, and the client later confirmed that this was a very accurate sensing. So it seems to me extremely evident that communication is about far, far more than the words that are being spoken.

Another example occurs to me. At an international gathering of person-centred folk, the idea emerged of delegates initially speaking in their first language and only *afterwards* having their words translated into English (rather than phrase by phrase). People spoke in several languages. With most delegates *I didn't understand a word that they said*, and for a few I understood at best the meaning of only a smattering of words. Yet I sure as hell *could* sense what they were *feeling* – and pretty accurately, too. Interestingly enough, for me the translations that followed tended to lack the emotive content which was expressed by the original speaker. Maybe you could try watching the television or a video with the sound muted. You might not hear a single word, yet my guess is that you will accurately perceive many of the emotions being expressed – perhaps largely through facial expression, gesture, bodily signals, and so on – so maybe these aspects of communication could be considered as the nature of 'non-verbal' signals. Or you could try listening to a tape and just focus on the *words* or, better still, look at a transcript of a tape and then listen to the tape, focusing on the *sounds*. Quite often, in my experience, the sounds impart information that the words do not, and this might illustrate the nature of 'paraverbal' communication.

And it does not stop there! A client who is extremely anxious might speak very rapidly. He or she might not use the word 'anxious', yet the rate of their speech might be communicating anxiety. Loudness of speech could be communicating anger, quietness might indicate feeling low or exhausted, and so on, and so on.

Thus my process of absorbing is in part about a seeing and hearing beyond the words that are spoken.

7 I'm confused. Are you saying that the client-centred therapist is somehow detached, somehow objectively absorbing and analysing – or processing, if you prefer – all of these sights and sounds?

No, that's not what I'm trying to communicate. It's interesting to me, because for many years I would experience a heated reaction to words like 'objective' in the belief that 'objective' symbolises 'cold', 'dispassionate', 'clinical' or whatever. To me, client-centred therapy is *involved* and *compassionate* and *subjective* and *warm* and . . . It is *in*-volved because I am really trying to be 'in there' with the client. Yet I realise as I speak that I am feeling some surprise at my lack of a strong reaction to the word 'objective' that I once would have felt. I think this is because the words 'subjective' and 'objective' have come to have less and less meaning and relevance for me. They both feel like the extremes of a linear scale, and my experience is that life ain't like that. Perhaps just as Rogers felt pretty passionately about the artificiality of separating *above the neck* and *below the neck*, believing rather that we are (potentially at least) whole persons, so I feel that this apparent need we have to be purely one thing or another is nonsense. Perhaps being a *whole person* doesn't mean being *wholly this* or *wholly that* – it could mean that the whole is comprised of many gradational aspects. So maybe I don't need to ferret out whether I am being *wholly objective* or *wholly subjective*. Maybe I can be a composite of many, many different attributes.

I know I have used the word *absorbing* a lot. Maybe another word to describe my process could be *immersing*. I feel as if I am immersing myself in my client's world of feelings and meanings. Although, to quote Rogers, I keep a sense of self about me (not losing the 'as if' quality of empathy), this hardly equates, for me, to the notion of objectivity. I want to say, too, and with some passion, that nor is this a *passive* process. Not only am I *trying really hard* to absorb and immerse myself in the world of my client, but also I will strive to communicate something of what I have sensed. It feels very *active* to me, far from passive.

8 You said that you regretted the focus on words . . .

Yes. And by this I mean that, for instance, I find it bizarre that 'the powers that be' consider it desirable – or even a requirement – for someone embarking on counselling diploma training to have completed counselling skills training. Now don't get me wrong, I think that counselling skills courses can be invaluable – there are many people for whom the implementation of counselling skills is their end aim, and that's great in my view. It is also very worthwhile, in my opinion, for people to have the opportunity to explore the mainstream therapeutic approaches prior to making as informed a choice as is possible of which diploma course to pursue. Yet over and over again my experience on diploma courses is that many trainees have spent at least the first term or two *unlearning* skills – and a process of *unlearning* the old alongside *learning* the new can be extremely problematic for many.

Oh gosh – this self-referencing is getting a bit embarrassing! I wrote another article called *How Do You Do* (I was really pleased with that title!), the gist of which was that in 'non-directive' counselling skills training, a kind of stock response would be 'How do you feel about that?'. Now it seems to me that 'How do you feel about that?' (hence the *How Do . . .* part of the title I like) is a perfectly good, non-directive (up to a point – the focus is on feelings), open-ended *response*. Yet if I am *communicating* empathy, my communication is more likely to be charac-terised by 'You feel sad' or 'You're really angry', or whatever (hence the *You Do . . .* part of the title). Note, too, the differentiation between a *response* (to a client's *words*, more often than not) and a *communication* (of sensing a client's moment-to-moment experiencing).

This focus on *words* is perhaps even more stark when it comes to *paraphrasing*, *summarising* and, Carl Rogers forbid, *reflecting*. It seems to me that the *process* is that many counselling skills trainees *have to focus on words* in order to be able to log and recall them for the purpose of paraphrasing, summarising, reflecting or whatever. And in the process of having to concentrate on the spoken word in order to be able to demonstrate specific skills and techniques, they very often miss out on the full depth and richness of what is passing between two people. So while I think that the implementation of skills certainly has its place, I am not convinced that such training is particularly helpful when it comes to a process of becoming client-centred.

So in general it would seem that most of *my* words thus far have not been about words – and for me this is significant. Perhaps now we can turn to the words themselves.

Of course the words that a client speaks are important. *Of course* it is important that I absorb and am able to remember a good proportion of the words that have been spoken. My point thus far has been that there is far, far more to communication than words alone. It almost seems helpful to think in terms of *essence* – and perhaps *essential*, too. Am I able somehow to distil the *essence* of what a client is communicating? What are the *essential* ingredients of a client's experiencing? As I said earlier, I remember watching a video of Carl Rogers in action, and he commenced one communication with 'I gather . . .', which I really liked. It triggered for me the idea that my process when I am striving to empathise is one of *gathering*. I am a *gatherer*, an *absorber*, of *all* of the elements of client communication. And if there is a whole universe of communication to absorb, maybe the words only represent one solar system. Within that system there may well be a very significant sun that casts light, or there may be significant planets, yet that solar system is only a part of the whole universe.

I might mention, too, that Rogers was interested in the process of finding the *right* words. Choose a word and look it up in a thesaurus. You now have a list of several words, all with very similar meanings. Yet when clients describe something, only *one* – just one – of those words seems to fit exactly. And you can *see* clients very obviously *referencing themselves* in order to sense, feel and think which word is the precise symbol of what they mean. Hit on the right word first time and hey – accurate empathy! Hit on one of the others, in a humble, flexible way, and clients experience your striving to empathically understand – and they will soon put you right if the relationship is one in which they feel free to do so.

9 You seemed to suggest that 'How do you feel about that?' wasn't entirely non-directive, because it focused on feelings. Could you say more about that?

I'd be delighted to! I have also spoken (and written) a few times about feelings *and meanings*, and this links with the word thing, too. Carl Rogers wrote that the *instant* we become aware of or perceive something, we attach a *meaning* to that awareness or perception. So if I just focus on the *words*, I might miss the *feelings and meanings* that lie 'behind' the words, or 'underneath' the words, or *inform* the words, or whatever. In other words (hah!), if I focus only on what is voiced (in order to paraphrase, reflect, or whatever), I run the very real risk of not sensing 'underlying' feelings or meanings.

Part of my agenda here is to try to dispel the myth that seems to have arisen about client-centred therapy (or the person-centred approach) being all to do with *feelings* – *because that is simply not true*. Read Rogers and you will quickly discover that he was consistent throughout his life, both in his writing and in his practice, about linking feelings *and meanings*. In his book *A Way of Being*, Carl wrote passionately about the artificial distinction that we make between 'head' and 'gut' (above the neck and below the neck, as he put it). If we are to be *whole* persons – that is, if I am to engage as one whole person with another whole person – then let us move away from yet another example of linear extremes –

head and gut! Feelings and personal meanings interweave; there is an incredibly rich flow between and among feelings and meanings.

10 What are your views on internal and external frames of reference?

I think that they may be useful concepts on the journey towards an empathic way of being when with clients, clarifying the difference between my world view (including my view of myself) and yours. And I guess that for me, when I am with a client what is internal and what is external is *usually* fairly clear – I think that I am relatively aware of what is 'my stuff' and what is 'the client's stuff'. The idea of a common frame of reference interests me, too, as I have already said.

11 You mean that there is a third frame of reference?

Oh yes! If you picture the 'Two Circles' diagram that Rogers used to illustrate and summarise the Nineteen Propositions (*Client-Centred Therapy* 1951, front cover and pp. 526–7) . . . you are seeing two circles, side by side – yes? So, using this format, the client's *internal* frame of reference would be in the left-hand-side segment, the therapist's frame of reference (that is, a frame of reference *external* to the client) would be in the right-hand-side segment, and the overlap would represent their *common* frame of reference. Thinking *only* in terms of internal and external frames of reference feels too rigid to me, too extreme and too linear. There is how you see the world, how I see the world, how we see the world, a pre-existing world of meanings (and feelings), the world that is becoming (new meanings, meanings in a process of being formed), and so on.

12 Did Carl Rogers write or say anything about this, or is this all your own thinking?

Some of both, I guess. There is Merleau-Ponti who I mentioned earlier, too. In fact there are many, many resources. As for Carl Rogers, when he wrote Proposition Seven in *Client-Centered Therapy* he mentioned that the experience and perceptions of others have counterparts in our own experience, and that these counterparts can be used as tentative guides. Thus when a client speaks of anger, for instance, I too have experienced anger, and although I need to be constantly aware that the client's feelings and meanings are 'unique' to that individual, it would also be naive, it seems to me, not to acknowledge that without some form of shared frame of reference there would be little if any communication.

So I can, perhaps, use my own frame of reference as a tentative guide into your frame of reference. I can also use our common frame of reference as a tentative guide into your frame of reference. On a simplistic level, we would probably all agree that a particular object is what can be called a chair, so 'chair' falls within our common frame of reference. However, we need to be aware that the chair has many properties that constitute its 'chairness', and that we shall not perceive the chair identically. For instance, one person might perceive shape first, another colour, another the material of which it is made, or whatever. I'm not sure that picking on a chair is necessarily the best example, but I hope that you are catching some of the sense of what I mean. And what the chair *means* to each of us might vary. For most of us, it probably goes no further than something to sit upon. Yet what if I was bound to a similar chair during a horrific assault, or it reminds me of my mother's chair, and my mother died recently, or something like that? So there is something about humility and remaining tentative. On the one hand, it may be reasonable to assume a probability that we do understand each other when we say 'chair', but on the other hand, we need to continually perception-check if we are striving towards empathic understanding.

So if as therapist I identify something as clearly 'my own stuff' – that is, 'stuff' from a frame of reference that is *external* to the client – then it follows that it is unlikely to have any place in the counselling room. If what emerges clearly belongs to the client – that is, from a frame of reference that is *internal* to the client – then it clearly has every significance to therapy. Sometimes, though, things seem to emerge from the space between us – from the hyphen of the I–thou relationship, if you will. I have come to trust what emerges in that space more and more, but then I also do a lot of exploring of such issues in my writing, my personal reflecting, and in supervision.

13 Did you mention memory as part of the internal frame of reference of the client? Doesn't that seem more like psychoanalytic thinking?

I want to be accurate here – can I just quickly look something up? This is the 1959 paper that Carl wrote, in which he gives us lots of definitions. Ah, here it is. I quote:

> *Internal frame of reference.* This is all of the realm of experience which is available to the awareness of the individual at a given moment. It includes the full range of sensations, perceptions, meanings, and memories, which are available to consciousness.
>
> (Rogers 1959: p. 210)

So the instant we perceive something we attach a meaning to it. When we speak of the *here and now* or of *immediacy*, our *current* experiencing includes any *past* experiencing (feelings and meanings) that have relevance to the here and now. So while the client-centred therapist does not *direct* the client to focus on past experience (or to then *analyse* that past experience), it is of course true that feelings and meanings gathered along the way may well pertain to current experiencing – and if the therapist is to grasp the intricacies and depth of current client experiencing, this understanding may well include the history that clients bring into *now*.

14 I've had two or three clients now, all of them male, and I just can't seem to get through their cognition and into their feelings. What can you say about that?

Okay . . . I think that I have a few thoughts about that. Let me see . . . I feel a reaction inside of me so that I know I have an agenda again, something I feel quite passionate about. Let me try to access this. It is that I want to try to dispel what seems to be a fairly popular myth that client-centred therapy is all about *feelings*. It isn't, as I have already said. Rogers wrote, for instance (I'm sorry that I'm repeating myself – it feels important), that every time we perceive something we instantly attach a meaning to it. And the meanings have importance, as do our perceptions, feelings and memories. There is something about *wholeness*. It reminds me of those who say that 'So long as I can be client-centred, why should I need to know theory?'. These same people will often talk about being whole persons or meeting clients as whole persons, or whatever. Yet *theory is an integral part of the wholeness of client-centred therapy*, and any reading of Rogers makes this crystal clear. How can I claim to be a whole person engaging with another whole person while at the same time dismissing an integral part of the whole of the approach that I claim to belong to?

Anyway, to get back to the point, I would want to be cautious about labelling a client as 'cognitive' or 'all head and no feeling', or whatever. Another issue that Carl Rogers was passionate about was this artificial differentiation that we make between feeling and thought. Read the part of *A Way of Being* where Rogers refers to Vincent Hanna and you will see what I mean. I feel passionate about this, too – it is yet another example, as I see it, of extreme and linear categorising, and it simply doesn't fit my experiencing of myself or others. So often people (including me) say 'I feel . . .' when what follows seems more like a thought, for instance. Well, that might just be language and pedantic, yet it does seem to me that there has been a trend in some client-centred circles to place more emphasis and value on feelings, to the detriment of meanings. And I think that this is a most regrettable trend, and one that Carl would have been hesitant to follow. In any case, how can I claim to regard you *unconditionally* if I value your feelings above your thoughts or, as I prefer, your personal meanings?

So if I am faced with an apparently 'cognitive' or 'heady' client, then maybe one of the first things I will want to explore is my own value system, to check out the authenticity of my unconditional positive regard. Thus there are real links with both congruence and unconditional positive regard here, it seems to me. I am also reminded (with, I confess, not a little embarrassment) of a client of mine from a few years back. A bit like the questioner, I felt frustrated that I could not get past all of his 'head stuff' and into his feelings. How I flinch now when I hear myself saying that! As if somehow I've got to apply this crowbar to get into a client's feelings! And even if my crowbar is wrapped in fluffy cotton wool, it is hardly client-centred! *Prizing* (with a 'z') *not prising* (with an 's') is a catchphrase I've come up with. Anyway, I took a tape of this client to supervision. To my eternal chagrin, after about ten minutes my supervisor stopped the tape and said something like 'Well, to me that was full of feeling'. This was an extremely salutary lesson for me to learn, and it is one that has stayed with me. What I had spectacularly failed to recognise was that my client was talking about his *feelings* in a *cognitive* way.

Another example comes to mind. Early in counsellor training (or in counselling skills development), a client begins – in a flat, steady, toneless voice and with an expressionless face and body – to say something like:

> Well, I've just discovered I am terminally ill, my partner has been laid off and our house is to be repossessed, and the cat was run over . . .

And the counsellor replies:

> How do you feel about that?

You can laugh, but it happens! For the sake of the point I am trying to make, we can say that there were no verbal, non-verbal or paraverbal clues to emotional content. Yet the client expects us to *infer* feeling. That is why people laugh –

because it seems absurd that the counsellor would not *infer feelings*. So maybe here is another clue about how to experience empathy. Perhaps this links to what Rogers meant when he wrote about empathic inference.

It seems to me that there is a tendency in client-centred circles to veer away from such discussion and exploration, because 'inference' gets equated with *analysis*, or *interpretation*, or *diagnosis*, or whatever – so best to avoid them. There is another possible example of our value base. I feel sure that words such as 'intuition' are somehow much more acceptable than 'inference', and I really think that this is a great shame, because sometimes I think that we miss out on exploring our processes as a consequence of such p-c p-c (person-centred political correctness!). Yet if I am to engage as a whole person, and if I have a capacity for inference, might not that capacity have a part to play? And if I can remain humble – that is, retain a sense of tentative humility – if I continually engage in a process of perception checking, might not this be another strand in the process of empathising?

To get back to our 'heady' client, then – first of all, can I experience acceptance? Can I value 'headiness' just as I value emotions, perhaps especially given an awareness that, at times at least, 'head' can be 'gut in disguise'? That doesn't feel right – it might be true, yet maybe I can value 'headiness' for precisely what it is (intellect, or brains, or whatever). Do I have to relegate someone's intellect to lower divisions, being interested only in the premier league of feelings, yet kid myself (and therefore con clients) into believing that I am being unconditional? Can I remain client-centred, thereby not utilising my crowbar to get at feelings? Can I gather whether my client might actually be talking about or alluding to feelings, yet in a cognitive way?

It seems to me, too, that other clients whom I have experienced as 'heady' have been using their intellect as a *defence* against their feelings. That's okay! If a client needs to protect himself (or herself, although I note the gender implications in the question) then that is their process in the moment. Rather than trying to prise my way into feelings, why not prize the individual? I may or may not communicate something of my sensing of their defensiveness, and that may or may not loosen up the expression of feelings. Yet I do not have any aim in mind other than to come as close as I can to being the core conditions of client-centred therapy.

So with a 'heady' client, it seems to me that if I can strive to authentically experience unconditional positive regard and empathic understanding, and the client is able to perceive this from me, then many things are both possible and, indeed, predictable. To stray from *being* client-centred makes client-centred *process* an impossibility, and would result in something that I predict would be very different in many respects.

15 How does all of this relate to what I've read about 'cognitive' and 'affective' empathy?

Well, I wouldn't want to dismiss those terms out of hand, as I guess that there are contexts within which they could be helpful. For example, if I am going through a transcript of a session with a client, I might want to make use of certain 'tools' or strategies that help me to explore how I was in that session. Many trainers say that 'cognitive empathy' is about understanding *meanings*, and affective empathy is about resonating with *feelings*. Well, okay, although I have already mentioned the artificiality of such harsh and linear distinctions. Nevertheless, it might prove helpful in terms of me exploring whether I could identify any predominant trends within me within the session. For instance, if I discover that I was relating mostly to meanings at the expense of engaging with feelings (or vice versa), why was that?

I suppose that I have to say, too, that in my experience as a trainer the idea of 'cognitive empathy' has not proved too useful. I can recall several instances where this kind of understanding has really been 'from the outside' – almost as if the trainee therapist is observing the client and understanding that they are feeling something and maybe why, too. Yet it somehow lacks the rich profundity of really getting into the client's world of feelings and meanings. Does 'inside out' as compared with 'outside in' make sense? Maybe this links with Carl Rogers differentiating between understanding *about* and understanding from *within* a client's frame of reference.

16 It reminds me of the 'You – because –' exercise we did on our skills course. Is this what you mean?

Yes, I think so – nice example (he said in a non-evaluative way!). This is often presented as 'You feel – because – ', as in 'You feel angry because this situation is unfair'. The 'You feel angry' part is presented as affective empathy and the 'because this situation is unfair' as cognitive empathy, or understanding. Put the two together and hey presto – empathic understanding! Yet this feels somewhat shallow to me. Again, I don't mean to be dismissive as I'm sure that this kind of empathic understanding has its place, either in itself or as part of a journey towards other ways of being empathic. But it somehow feels 'clever', 'dispassionate' or 'detached' when compared with the incredible experience of almost becoming the other person – without losing the 'as if' quality, of course! There is a title in that somewhere – 'On Becoming Your Client' perhaps! So it occurs to me that the 'You – because – 'type of empathic understanding, albeit somewhat formulaic, has a richness that simply reflecting, paraphrasing or posing open-ended, non-directive questions does not have, yet at the same time it lacks the richness that I hope I have described. And remember that Carl did distinguish between understanding *about* and 'truly' understanding from *within* the client's frame of reference.

17 Wasn't there talk of Rogers going to include intuition as a seventh condition, or a fourth core condition?

Well, if there wasn't, it would seem as if there is right now! My understanding is that there *has* been some talk of intuition being added as a seventh condition, or a fourth 'core' condition, but not by Carl Rogers! It is true that, especially later in his life, Carl became very interested in the intuitive aspects of his empathy, although my understanding is that Rogers looked at intuition under the umbrella of empathy, so to speak.

18 So do you have views about intuition?

Of course! Intuition fascinates me. I have increasingly come to trust my intuition, too, although yet again I strive to maintain a kind of tentative humility. I have not to date encountered an explanation of this intuitive capacity that I have come to trust, so I tried to formulate my own.

I recall meeting with a client for the first time. He described his experience of a one-night stand and how rejected and worthless he felt on being spurned at college the next day. At one point I said something like 'And this feels so much more raw because this person was another guy', and I remember feeling *astonished* – it was as if the words just kind of 'popped into my head' and it felt as if I wasn't at all in control of my own process. It felt scary, almost, and certainly very bewildering. Yet after a pause, the client said 'You've just saved several weeks of therapy – but how on earth did you know?'.

I listened to a tape of this session many times, and began to formulate a theory around my own intuitive process. I think that I should perhaps stress at this point that to me this feels like an extreme example of my intuition, yet it was significant in shaping my thinking. What I discovered through listening to the tape was that the client had been very careful about using gender-free terminology – for example, several times he said things like 'the other person', or 'they', or 'them', or whatever. Not once had he used a gender-specific word. At the time I was not *consciously* aware of this, yet my belief now is that at some level just 'behind', or 'beneath' or 'at the edge of' full awareness, my brain had somehow 'clocked' this careful choosing of words – not just once but in a sequence. In retrospect, it feels as if as this sequence accumulated it eventually became strong enough to break through into awareness, and *that* was the intuitive moment. For me, this explanation of this particular instance feels right. I am not convinced that such an explanation applies to *all* intuitive moments, though. As I speak I am wondering if there might be links between what I was saying about empathic inference and empathic guessing and intuition, too.

I want to return more directly to trying to explain my process of empathising. It seems to me that another vital aspect is the sixth necessary and sufficient condition – that the client perceives, at least to a minimal degree, the unconditional positive regard and empathic understanding of the therapist. What a tragic waste if I utilise my senses to try to sense what the client is experiencing moment by moment, yet then do not communicate anything of the outcomes of my efforts! You know, again it seems to me that this is a critical point in differentiating between the implementation of counselling skills and being an empathic therapist. When being at my best empathically, I think that *I use very little of my capacity in thinking about what I am going to say next.* This feels very, very different to me from trying to identify, store and recall words for the purpose of paraphrasing, summarising, reflecting, or whatever. It also feels much more deeply immersed in the *client's* world of perceptions, feelings and meanings than offering an open-ended, non-directive question. Rather, the words seem to flow.

In really trying to *gather* and *absorb* the client's feelings and meanings, and then offering the fruits of my harvesting, I need not be too concerned about the quality of storage and recall, formulation and so on. Rather, I am striving to communicate my striving to empathise and understand. I can honestly say that thoughts about *implementing skills* (such as 'reflecting') just never, ever enter my head. It is hard to explain properly. At my best, I am just so immersed in trying to experience the feelings and meanings of the other person that when I speak it is as if I *were* that other person – or at least as if I am some close approximation to that other person. It is *incredibly* unlikely that this other person is thinking about reflecting my words back to me, or paraphrasing my words, or whatever – so it is equally unlikely that I will be! Even if a client feels stuck, or numb, then my striving is to experience what their numbness feels like and what feeling stuck means to them, and whatever will flow, will flow – or not, as the case may be. I am striving to be *in there with them*, not intending to pull them out, or move them on, or whatever. I think that sometimes counsellors do not enter the numbness, 'stuckness' or stasis of clients because not to try to pull them out or move them on somehow feels like abandoning them to their hopelessness, but far from it. I cannot be *really in there* with someone if I am hell-bent on trying to get them moving.

19 I'm sorry to disagree with the last questioner, but I was told that Rogers was going to include spirituality as the fourth core condition. Is this true?

Again, to the best of my knowledge, the answer is no, this is not true. I feel concerned and somewhat suspicious about how such rumours arise. I suspect that they say more about the people who would like to see spirituality incorporated into client-centred therapy or the person-centred approach than they do about Carl Rogers. I have no particular quibble with the therapist who is spiritual – and I guess it's a very personal, individual thing anyway. Perhaps of greater importance is therapist *congruence* – if I *am* spiritual I need to in some way *be* spiritual, and if I'm not, I won't be. I do feel concerned, though, when people say '*Carl* was going to make spirituality a condition', without backing it up. Show me where Carl said or wrote that – yes?

Carl expressed caution about even using the word 'spirituality', and this would seem to include a couple of things. First, he was eager to avoid religious connotations and connections, for if he *did* use the word, he meant it in a non-religious way. Second, he commented that the word 'spirituality' meant so many different things to so many different people that there was a lack of clarity in meaning. Carl did clarify his own meaning, though. He spoke and wrote of how, when being deeply empathic, it almost felt like an altered state of consciousness, and that he would experience a kind of connectedness between his own 'spirit' or 'essence' and the 'spirit' or 'essence' of the client. He talks with Gay Barfield about this on the *Empathy: an Exploration* video from 1985, and it is very clear to me that even if couched in terms of 'transcending the everyday' or 'altered states of consciousness', his thinking nevertheless falls very definitely within the realms of empathic understanding – an *existing* therapist condition.

So no, I know of no evidence that Carl was thinking of any new conditions, spiritual or intuitive or otherwise.

Incidentally, Carl also said in his 'A Way of Meeting Life' interview (Rogers, 1984: p. 2) that he originally had no interest in a notion so vague as a 'self' but that he researched it because client after client referred to it. If he had another lifetime and clients perpetually referred to spirit, then that's the way he would go – and he recognised a trend towards the more spiritual and was certainly open to it.

20 What exactly does 'the client receives, at least to a minimal degree' actually mean? You mentioned this just now

Now there's a question! One of my worries about training in client-centred therapy is that we don't really have any locally, nationally or internationally agreed measure of what 'minimal' means.

I think that it could be helpful to link the first and sixth necessary and sufficient conditions here – 'two persons are in contact' (or 'psychological contact' if you prefer) and 'the client receives the unconditional positive regard and empathic understanding of the therapist' (at least, as you said, to a minimal degree). With regard to being in contact, Rogers wrote about 'contact' as meaning that the therapist makes a significant difference in the perceptual (or phenomenal) field of the client. So from this we might infer (or intuit!) that 'receiving to a minimal degree' is to do with being heard, maybe to do with a degree of understanding, and so on. In the video I have just mentioned where Carl Rogers and Gay Barfield discuss empathy, and in another video where Carl takes a question from the audience on empathy, what emerges is the idea of *reciprocal empathy* – and that makes sense to me. In other words (and the video audience seemed a little surprised by this idea when Carl voiced it), *we rely upon our clients to empathise with and understand our attempts to empathise with and understand them*. This might go some way towards clarifying not only the notion of 'contact', but also the notion of the client receiving, at least to a minimal degree, the empathy of the therapist.

It also reminds me of a question in the CORE (Clinical Outcomes in Routine Evaluation) forms, which are widely used in the UK within the NHS to try to measure the effectiveness of counselling. The therapist is asked to rate the 'psychological mindedness' of clients. I guess that one of the ways in which I might think about a client's 'psychological mindedness' is the degree to which he or she is able to receive my striving to empathise with and understand him or her – although I'm also aware as I speak that an exceptionally rigid self-structure might be linked, for me, with rating psychological mindedness at the lower end of the scale.

As this goes on, I realise that two perhaps separate issues are emerging for me. One is the nature of contact, and reciprocal empathy ('the client receives . . .'), and I feel okay about that. The other is this notion of 'minimal', and I don't feel okay about that. If, say, a trainee produces a transcript of a counselling session in which there are 25 counsellor communications, three of which demonstrate empathy and 22 of which do not, are we to say that 12% adequately evidences a 'minimal degree'? Probably not, yet in terms of simple arithmetic, my guess is that 12% could accurately be described as minimal. So can someone who is communicating empathy 12% of the time accurately describe themselves as client-centred? Or can we say that if *all* of a counsellor's communications involve a *minimal* degree of empathy – yet also major degrees of some other quality that falls outside the core conditions – they are client-centred? Or is the *client* the sole determinant of receiving to a minimal degree? Is it all about the client's 'psychological mindedness' or reciprocal empathy?

I'd like to quickly throw in another couple of ideas. I found it really liberating to hear Carl say (in the Radio Telefís Eireann Dublin interview) that rather than placing a condition upon oneself (he was actually talking about unconditional positive regard) – which leaves the self wide open to feelings of failure and inadequacy if the condition is not met – we can instead think in terms of being fortunate if the condition is met to some degree. I think that I am more likely to succeed with empathy if I view achieving it as a fortunate bonus, rather than striving to avoid failure. I also like the idea of some being better than none, and more being better than some. Again, I think that holding such a view is liberating, whereas striving to meet ideal conditions is almost bound to lead to failure. Too much empathy can be a bad thing, too. Carl wrote of counsellors who tried so hard to be empathic (in order to impress themselves or others) that they became insensitive to clients.

It seems to me that if the third, fourth and fifth necessary and sufficient conditions (congruence, unconditional positive regard and empathic under-standing on the part of the therapist) are met, then defining the *receiving* of these with reference to the *client* would seem to make some sense. At the same time, the second necessary and sufficient condition is that the client is incongruent, so we might ask what degree of denial and/or distortion of our empathic commun-ications is acceptable!

I wonder if this links in any way with Carl's changes to the sixth necessary and sufficient condition. Sometimes Carl wrote of the therapist *communicating* uncon-ditional positive regard and empathy, and at other times he wrote about the client *receiving* unconditional positive regard and empathy. My understanding is that Carl preferred the client *receives* version on the grounds that the therapist *communicating* empathic understanding could represent a regrettable pathway towards the teaching of skills, something he was most keen to avoid. So maybe there is no link there. However, we could make one if we so choose.

21 What are your views on therapist self-disclosure and the process of empathy, or empathising? And earlier you mentioned material that arises from the hyphen in the I–thou relationship . . .

I guess that it will come as no surprise that my views on therapist self-disclosure are much the same as those that Carl Rogers expressed on many occasions. Let me try the kind of 'glib, by the book' response first.

Rogers said that if a therapist experienced a personal feeling or thought *persistently*, then it probably belonged in the counselling relationship. Maybe we can break this down somewhat, though. What does 'persistent' mean? Two or three times in one session, or over a period of sessions, or what? Rogers was very clear about congruence not meaning that the therapist 'impulsively blurts out every passing feeling', so there is another link with the idea of a feeling or thought being *persistent* or occurring over a prolonged period of time. So it is my view that if *over a period of time* (and for me that would be perhaps two or three sessions) a feeling, thought or meaning is *persistent*, then I have plenty of time to reflect and explore along the way. Now let us assume that I have decided, either as a result of self-reflecting or as an outcome of supervision, that this persistent feeling or thought *does* belong in the therapeutic relationship. This does not mean that I will begin the next session with it! Nor will I be 'biding my time' until it comes up! If I introduce the feeling or thought, then the therapy is no longer client-centred and directed by the client. If I am simply 'treading water', eager for my opportunity, then I am not as fully present for the client as I could be. For me, this process is more about being open to sharing this persistent feeling or thought *should it occur again naturally in the course of the therapy*. I trust that if there *is* any significance and relevance to my persistent feeling or thought, then I can anticipate that it will occur again as a matter of course. I need be in no hurry! And I am open to the feeling or thought not recurring, too.

As I think about it, I realise that what I have just said is not entirely truthful. I think, if I'm honest, that there have been times when a feeling or thought has been persistent within a single therapy session, and that I have voiced such feelings or thoughts on occasions. As I said that, I wondered if there might be a further link with intuitive moments, or with empathic guessing or inference. If there is persistence within one therapy session, I think that I tend to perform an 'internal check' in order to satisfy a few questions, such as 'Is this my stuff or the client's?' and 'Am I able to access unconditional positive regard and empathy to the full?', and so on. If my feeling or thought seems to be acting as a barrier to empathic understanding, then I need to find a way to remove it. This *may* mean voicing it. It might also mean that I 'make it recede' and empathy comes to the fore. I like the visualisation of a sound recording mixing desk, with several sliding volume controls – I can lower the volume of my own thought or feeling and pump up the empathy!

We could also look at how the therapist's persistent feeling or thought is introduced to the counselling relationship. Rogers said that he would usually accompany any such communication *with his own feelings or thoughts about his disclosure*. I wonder if I can think of an example of this. I know that at times I might say something like 'I'm not at all sure where this is coming from, yet . . .' or 'I'm a little unsure whether I've understood you correctly – there would seem to be something around . . .'. Maybe they are not such good examples. I feel a little reluctant to share this, because I think that it is a real exception rather than some kind of 'rule' that I follow. I remember one client I found myself disliking pretty intensely. This feeling persisted. In the end (and after a great deal of agonising and exploring), I voiced something of how I did not look forward to meeting with him. In some respects, he seemed quite relieved to have this out in the open. Clients ain't daft! They sense things. It transpired that on this occasion my disclosure that I was really struggling to experience unconditional positive regard was quite helpful both to the client and to the therapeutic relationship. My disclosure was not said in a blaming way, and I was very careful to own my words (while at the same time being aware that no matter how much I own my words, that isn't necessarily how they will be heard). Carl Rogers also felt that the owning of words was important. There is a difference between saying 'I am experiencing boredom' and 'You are a boring person', although I still think that the former is often nevertheless heard as the latter – one excellent reason for caution around self-disclosing, in my view. Anyway, it turned out that this particular client had no friends at all, and was 'disliked by everybody' – that was his problem as he saw it. So having someone voicing their experiencing of dislike, yet in a compassionate and respectful way (doesn't that sound strange?) actually gave him an opportunity to explore how he was experienced by others – the real 'nitty-gritty' of why he was there in the first place.

I feel uncomfortable now. I do want to stress that this example is exceptional, in my experience. I do not regularly experience dislike for clients and then voice it!

I have just thought of another example, but it feels pretty exceptional again. Some years ago I recall a client who I experienced as powerfully exuding two things from every single pore in her body – sex and vulnerability. It was not just sex, but 'raw sex' – a real sexy sexiness. And not just vulnerability, but a really raw fragility. Now bearing in mind that I was at that time being investigated under a professional complaints procedure, I understandably felt that I had to be pretty careful about anything I said. As a professional sanction, I was required to change to an accredited supervisor, who was psychodynamic. 'What are you worried about?', he said, 'I frequently say things like "I'm having sexual thoughts about you and I'm wondering where they're coming from" – it's all part of transference and counter-transference'. Thanks a lot – very helpful! Fortunately, I always tape recorded sessions with this client, and I think that this was a significant factor in my eventually 'going for it' and voicing something of how I experienced her. Let me take a step back a moment. One outcome for me was that I realised that a simultaneous mixture of vulnerability and sex was a pretty powerful cocktail for me to experience. I reflected on this a great deal, including exploring my issues in personal therapy. I learned a great deal about myself and grew through this process. So to an extent, I can say that my experiencing of this client represented 'my stuff', and I don't think that stuff that is purely mine has any place in therapy (at least, not when I am the therapist!). On the other hand, there was something about this client. It *was she* who was exuding the sex and vulnerability, not me. It was not 'my fantasy' – I was absorbing signals *from her*. So clearly there was also an element that was not simply 'my stuff'. I felt some kind of 'charge' or 'energy' in the space between us. I was pretty confident that she experienced this, too, although I was less confident as to how conscious this experiencing was to her. Anyway, in the end I 'went for it'. It was very scary for me and it felt as if my only security was the tape recording. As it happened, it turned out to be good. It was therapeutic. This client had repeatedly experienced dissatisfying liaisons and constantly asked herself the question 'Why me?'. I want to be absolutely clear here that we didn't get into some kind of 'she was asking for it' scenario. However, what did unfold was a real opportunity for this client to explore how the 'signals' that she emitted might have consequences for her. In other words, she became more self-aware and as a result became more empowered, more able to make choices. I'm not sure that I've done justice here, yet I hope that you catch something of my meaning.

You know, given that to me both of the above examples feel exceptional, you can probably conclude from this that only very rarely do I personally self-disclose. Like Rogers, I believe that being congruent or 'transparent' or 'genuine' does not mean 'impulsively blurting out every passing feeling' or that 'anything goes'. I also believe that there is an absolute, direct link between 'transparency' and the degree to which unconditional positive regard and empathic understanding are deeply embedded as natural aspects of my way of being. By this I mean that impulsively blurting out every passing feeling does not necessarily have to mean that I am incongruent in that moment. However, to me it *would* mean that I have yet to deeply incorporate unconditional positive regard and empathy in my therapeutic way of being. It might mean that perhaps I have more self-exploring to undertake, too.

Can I think of a less extreme example? Let us say that a client 'has a go at me', saying that I don't really understand and, after all, that I am being paid to just sit and listen. One of my inner reactions is of righteous indignation and defensiveness (this is an affront to my self-concept, so I feel a need to protect it), so I gently let the client know that truly I *am* trying really hard to enter their world of feelings and personal meanings. Am I being congruent? No, because I am denying myself access to those respectful and empathic capacities that I hold so dear. Okay, so I respect this client and empathise with the frustration, or anger, or feelings of hopelessness that are being expressed. Am I being congruent now? No, because I am denying myself access to my feelings of indignation, and they are real enough, too. Congruence means allowing myself access to *all* significant parts of me in the moment, and making choices based on this accessing. Thus, for me, *any self-disclosure involves choice on my part* – what I will choose to disclose and what I will not choose to disclose, why and when and what . . .

I'm reminded of reading a transcript of an interview that Carl Rogers gave a month or two before he died. He was asked if he had any regrets. He replied that as he himself was a *disciplined* person, he had mistakenly assumed that other client-centred therapists were self-disciplined practitioners, too. He realised that this was far from always being the case, and he wished that he had placed greater emphasis on client-centred therapy being a disciplined approach. For me, the therapist who regularly self-discloses lacks the discipline to put the commitment to stay within the client's frame of reference fully into practice.

Having stated that Rogers believed that any *persistent* feeling or thought that arose within a therapeutic relationship probably belonged in that relationship, this reminds me a little of applying the 'Two Circles' diagram to frames of reference as we did earlier. There is 'material' that is clearly the client's, material that is clearly mine (these two would be in the outer segments), and material that has arisen between us (in the overlap segment, or in the hyphen of the I–thou relationship). I feel okay about voicing anything that is the client's or that has arisen in the space between us, yet I am more cautious about anything that is clearly in *my* segment. However, if it is persistent and I have checked it out, then I may well share it.

I guess that if I were to dredge up my most important agenda here, it would be about not 'letting it all hang out' and 'in your face' self-disclosing – this was never what was intended by 'transparency' or congruence or authenticity or being genuine. So I come back to the degree to which unconditional positive regard and empathic understanding are deeply embedded, and a self-aware way of being that does not deny or distort significant experiencing.

22 How does your process of empathising link with what Dave Mearns has written about configurations of self?

Hmm, well, I don't want to be disrespectful to Dave Mearns, but just to set the record straight, Carl Rogers used the term 'configurations of self' as early as 1959, so I don't think it is accurate to consider this term wholly as a creation of Dave's! Incidentally, Carl also said that he didn't *particularly* care for configurations of self theory, but that he was fine with those who did (he stated that he was more interested in the process of becoming than in somewhat fixed self-structures). Nevertheless, I personally find the idea of *configurations of self* pretty helpful, although whether or not the use I make of this theory is quite what was intended I do not know.

There are a couple of things that occur to me, and one of these is an issue that I am still in the process of working through, so it feels like unfinished processing to me.

The first issue (one that I feel is pretty sorted for me) concerns how helpful I find looking at configurations of self in supervision, specifically with a view to exploring the nature of my unconditional positive regard and empathic understanding. An example that I have used before is that of the client who self-injures. In this instance, there is a 'client self' who is doing the cutting, a 'client self' who is being cut, and a 'client self' who is 'overseeing' the action between the 'hurter' and the 'hurt'. Once a self (or a configuration of self) has been symbolised, it becomes a self-as-object – something identified, something named – something that can be broken down into its component parts and examined and explored. The self-as-process is doing the exploring. I find it helpful in supervision to explore the degree to which I am engaging with each of these aspects of the client's whole. For instance, I might discover that I feel somehow 'seduced' into empathising with the victim and the hurt, and as a consequence I may be neglecting the hurter or the self-as-process. Alternatively, I might believe that the hurter, the perpetrator, is more in need of the core conditions if change is to be generated, so the hurt and the processor become neglected. Or I might be so in awe of the client's motivation to change that I engage with the processor and neglect the hurter and the hurt. Whatever, what I appreciate is the opportunity – a framework or strategy, if you like – to explore the depth and extent of my engagement with clients. And if I discover that I am neglecting certain 'configurations of self' in a client's self-structure, I can also explore whether or not there might be links with configurations within my own self-concept. So I do find the notion of configurations of self very helpful as a strategy or process that I can use to try to maximise the extent to which the whole of me is open to the whole of the client, including maximising the unconditional nature of my positive regard and striving to ensure empathy with and understanding of all significant aspects of the client.

The second issue I'm not so sure about. I'm not so sure about it because it feels maybe directive, or it seems as if the therapist is taking the lead, or something, yet I don't want these thoughts to get too much in the way of exploring the issues. Let me stray into an anecdote. There is a large international gathering of person-centred people. Some are known to all (the 'big names', the 'A list'), others are known to many (the 'B list'), some are known to some (the 'C list', the 'minor celebrities'), and yet others are not known at all, or certainly did not feel known (the 'D list'). Some people were very evident – visible and speaking out. Others were somewhat hidden in the outer rings of the circles, saying nothing. I asked if Venya was present. Venya had come from Russia and we had exchanged emails but had never met 'in the flesh', so to speak. We connected. I later approached several people and engaged with them, and as a consequence they engaged with me and moved on to engage with others. There was another person from Poland, and I recall saying something like 'I realise that this is my need and I don't want to pressure you. I want to say that I feel I'm really missing out through not hearing you speak'. This person then spoke for some time – and in part expressed gratitude for feeling welcomed for the first time.

I thought about these experiences, and wondered whether such *community* processes might in any way be relevant to experiencing a group of configurations of self – a *community of selves* that make up a whole person. If I think about clients, there are certain self-aspects that are equivalent to 'A list celebrities' – being very visible and outspoken. There are also hidden, coy or silent aspects of self, and often a good many in between. Might these (or some of these) hidden or silent selves appreciate some kind of recognition or welcome? Might these selves be wondering whether or not it is safe to come out and play, and yearn for an invitation? I'm reminded of another international person-centred gathering at which the first few hours were spent negotiating seating arrangements. Many people engaged meaningfully with this (it triggered all kinds of feelings and thoughts about inclusion and exclusion, power and equality, for instance). Others tolerated the process, and two social workers who were interested in the person-centred approach left within the first 24 hours of what was a five-day meeting. Why? Because *they didn't know the rules*. They didn't know what to expect. Most of all, they didn't feel either acknowledged or welcomed. Could this apply to configurations of self within an individual's self-concept? If an aspect of self feels neglected, ignored or unwelcome, might it just go away?

I'm really not sure about this one. To welcome a self that is barely visible feels somewhat directive – no, it doesn't feel somewhat directive, it feels *directive*. Welcoming a barely visible self could be received by the client as ignoring, sabotaging or hijacking the self in full flow at that moment, for instance, and it is my choice to do so. Yet just before he died, Rogers reiterated (here I'm thinking of the chapter he wrote with Nat Raskin for *Current Psychotherapies*) that from time to time he would tentatively venture his sensing of feelings and personal meanings of which the client seemed only dimly aware, or even completely unaware – 'edge of consciousness' material. And it seems to me that such 'hidden' selves could be regarded as 'lurking at the edge of awareness'. I don't want to come across as too patronising or arrogant here, but I can honestly say that over the years my trust in venturing such tentative 'feelers' (tentative tentacles!) has grown somewhat. I have followed my client's lead when I have done so, and, whatever it sounds like, it has usually proved to be both relevant and helpful.

Perhaps I should also mention that, fairly often in fact, clients identify their own 'configurations of self' and want to explore them, sometimes also wanting to explore the nature of the inter-relationships between their selves. That is okay – they sing, I accompany.

I want to return to a more specific focus on my process of empathising, and say something about the links between empathic understanding, congruence and unconditional positive regard.

23 What, then, do you see as being the relationship between empathic understanding and congruence and unconditional positive regard?

I have a dim recollection that I said I would answer the question on therapist self-disclosure in two ways, and only answered it in the glib one. Maybe here is my opportunity to give the other version.

Let us assume that we are right at the start of a training course in client-centred therapy. Let us also assume for the moment that there is not a stunningly high degree of unconditional positive regard or empathic understanding being experienced or communicated – otherwise why the need to embark on a training programme? Now for me this does not have to mean that course members are necessarily being *incongruent*. However, it may well be that unconditional positive regard and empathic understanding are not as deeply embedded as fundamental and integral aspects of the self as they could be. For instance, if I respond to your communication with a 'This is how it is for me'-type response, this does not have to mean that I am denying or distorting anything.

My hope would be that as person-centred learning progresses, so unconditional positive regard and empathic understanding *do* become more deeply embedded as integral, fundamental and authentic aspects of the therapist. As this happens, so disclosure to clients from the internal frame of reference of the therapist becomes less and less likely. In other words, I am more likely to respond to your disclosure with an authentic attempt at letting you know that I am respectfully striving to understand your world of feelings and meanings.

Another way of saying this is that unless empathic understanding is authentic, it is less likely to be of value. At the same time, Rogers stated that the best way to communicate unconditional positive regard is via empathy.

24 Do you see each of the core conditions as having different relevance or importance to different phases of the therapeutic process?

Gosh – yes and no, I suppose! Now why did I say that?

I guess that the 'Yes' feels kind of heady – something about clients entering therapy being vulnerable, anxious and defensive. The theory – and my experi ence as both therapist and client – is that the client's receiving of unconditional positive regard serves to dissolve conditions of worth and serves to dissipate defensiveness. Very often it seems to me that unconditional positive regard features very highly in the early stages of therapy. Yet very often therapy moves into a real searching for meaning, and here maybe empathy and under-standing feel somehow more significant. Neither respect nor empathy are likely to be of much value if they lack authenticity, so I guess I'd see congruence as vital throughout.

Yet I have a strong 'No' response, too. This is based on the artificiality of breaking down the core conditions into component parts. I don't want to lose sight of the whole person. Although we break things down into manageable portions in order to digest them, let us not forget that a spark plug sure ain't the whole engine, and the car won't run if we don't put the motor back together again! So if we do take things apart in order to examine them, let's not forget to put them back together.

25 How do you empathise with silence, or the client who says very little? Is it true that the client-centred therapist should never be the one to break a silence?

How do I empathise with silence? Well, as I have said, there's far more to the universe of communication than just the solar system of the spoken word. Thus although in silence there is no *verbal* communicating, there might still be some paraverbal communication (such as sighing, or specific fast or slow or deep or shallow breathing) and lots of non-verbal communication. So I guess that mostly I use my eyes. For instance, facial expressions can tell us a great deal. I know that sometimes I shift my body shape to approximate to that of the client's in the hope that this will give me some insight into their possible sensations. Sometimes I might actually shift, and sometimes I just *imagine* sitting that way and what it would feel like. Sometimes I also stare at my hands or imagine my face being set in the same way. I don't have any rules or set techniques other than to strive to get into the client's world of feelings and meanings in whatever way feels appropriate at the time.

I recall someone asking Carl Rogers about the client who seemingly doesn't say very much, and he replied that *most* clients don't say very much! He reckoned that most clients say only a few things of central or deep significance in a therapy session. Some surround these significant disclosures with many other words, and some surround them with silence.

Where does 'The client-centred therapist should never be the one to break a silence' come from? Was it something you were told on your skills course? My guess is that this was justified on the grounds of not intruding into the client's space or something. Yes? Okay. 'Empathic guessing' and 'empathic inference' have been referred to a few times already. Rogers wrote about these in (among other places) a chapter called 'The Silent Young Man', and in the transcripts you will see that Carl Rogers broke just about every silence. So wherever the idea came from that client-centred therapists don't break silences, it didn't come from Rogers! I guess that not being intrusive would be based on a notion of respect for a client's space, which on the face of it sounds okay. Yet venturing an empathic guess could be respectful, too. Perhaps there could be something about maintaining and enhancing the 'two persons in contact' element through empathic inference as well. I would estimate that I probably speak first after half or more of the silences that I meet with in therapy, and almost always with some attempt at empathy – either empathic understanding if the non-verbal and paraverbal signals are fairly clear (for instance, I might say something like 'You're feeling really fidgety right now'), or with an empathic guess if the signals are less clear. Very occasionally I might even self-disclose! I have sometimes said something like 'I really can't sense with any accuracy what's going on for you right now, but I am interested if or when you're ready to speak . . .'.

There's something about this *how* to empathise that I feel uncomfortable with, at least sometimes. I think that this is about feeling okay with the core conditions being stipulated – it being necessary (and sufficient) to be congruent, respectful and empathic – yet feeling ill at ease when it comes to *stipulating* how. So the fact that Rogers broke nearly all silences doesn't have to mean that you should do so, too. And the fact that I break half or more of the silences doesn't mean that this has to be an objective for you. So by all means be authentically and respectfully empathic, but be so in your own way.

26 Do you ever not experience empathy, or experience a loss of empathy, and if so, what do you do about it?

Who, me? Of course not, never! Yes, of course I do. Maybe I can reframe the question to ask *why* I might not experience empathy, or *why* I might lose it. The first thought that occurs to me is that I might lose empathy if one of my own thoughts, feelings or sensations is getting in the way, in which case I need to deal with it. I have already talked about this – maybe whatever it is recedes as I pump up the empathy volume, or maybe I voice something. I find it more difficult to sustain empathy if I'm extremely tired or distracted, so I need to take care of myself if I'm striving to be fully present for clients.

It seems to me that a crucial factor here is therapist *self-awareness*. Sometimes loss of empathy feels quite sudden, a kind of surprised realisation – 'where did that go?'. In such instances it feels quite easy to become empathic once again. I simply refocus on striving to sense what the client is experiencing in this moment. At other times there is a kind of creeping, growing awareness of feeling less connected with either the client or my empathy, or with both, although again internal monitoring and accessing feels like the crucial factor in reconnecting.

Then there is the question of how to reconnect. Very often it really is as simple as turning my attention to what the client is feeling and what meanings might be present in the moment. There has been something in the background here that feels really embarrassing – 'aw shucks' and all that. I have a framed picture of Carl Rogers on my wall, and sometimes when I realise that I need to reconnect, I glance at it. This feels embarrassing because maybe it sounds like hero worship or something 'sad'. Well, I clearly have great admiration for Carl Rogers, but that's not it. The picture acts as a kind of instant trigger for me. To me, the picture symbolises what Carl stood for, like the necessity and sufficiency of the core conditions. So one quick glance and bam – it all comes flooding back! I believe that I can undertake this instant reconnecting with my capacity to strive to be the core conditions with or without a picture – it just happens to be there and it helps. I guess that almost anything could be used to symbolise the core conditions – a plant, the clock, the box of tissues, my own awareness, my mind . . .

So maybe something common to all of us is an awareness that empathy has been lost or is fading. However, *how* we reconnect with our empathic selves and our clients might be more personal.

27 Isn't there something about setting aside your own feelings and thoughts or, better still, shouldn't your baggage be left outside the room?

Not for me, no. To me, that doesn't make much sense. You look taken aback. Okay, let me try and explain. First of all I'm not entirely happy with the word 'baggage', as it doesn't exactly feel like unconditional acceptance – rather, it feels somewhat derogatory and dismissive. I'm sure we wouldn't dismiss a client's baggage so readily, so maybe we can afford ourselves the same respect that we offer to clients. Secondly, how is it possible to speak of therapists being *whole persons* in the relationship if they leave chunks of themselves outside? I'm reminded of the earlier theme about client-centred discipline, too – the discipline to live out my stated commitment to striving to be the therapist conditions, that includes staying within the client's frame of reference as much as I am able to. Also I wrote a piece relatively recently in which I came up with the idea of an empathy *muscle*. Don't use your empathy muscle and it will atrophy and wither. Use and exercise your empathy muscle regularly and it will easily be strong enough to carry baggage with no problem.

I don't mean to sound too abrupt, but it's late and I'm feeling a bit worn out. As we only have a few minutes left, I'd like to make copies of the article on 'Setting Aside Or Erupting?' available to those who would like to explore this theme further, which might make it more acceptable to move quickly on. Would that be okay?

28 I'm really interested in the use of imagery and metaphor. Do you use them?

Yes. I realise that I responded with a spontaneous and definite 'yes', yet it occurs to me that my use of imagery, analogy and metaphor is something that has very much grown over the years. I guess there might even have been a time when I didn't use them at all. Maybe I've grown in confidence, or something. Maybe I've just grown! Or I am growing . . . One thing I love is the diversity of commun-ication available to us. Why not exploit all of the rich ways of communicating at our disposal?

29 Can you give any examples?

Okay, I can think of two examples from the last couple of days that I feel quite pleased with! Now that's interesting – why do I say *'pleased'*? I guess it might sound as if I feel smug about having 'done my job well' or something, but that's not it. It might be *part* of it, but I think it's much, much more to do with feeling pleased with the reaction from the clients – like their response to me let me know that I really was with them in their world, and that feels really enriching, meaningful (to both of us) and worthwhile. Anyway, one client is a shop worker, and she had described (several sessions previously) how she would be at work and her mother would appear peering pleadingly through the front window, and just how difficult the client found this. This week she was reflecting on how her relationship *with herself* in relationship to her mother had changed over the course of her therapy. I recall saying something like:

> It doesn't feel like there are shutters or walls between you any more. It feels more like the glass shop window. Sometimes you just wave at her because you are very busy, and that feels okay now. Sometimes you are busy serving someone else, and it feels okay for mom to wait in the queue. Hell, sometimes you even shut up shop – and even that feels okay now, too.

The client became quite excited – it seemed as if I had captured her feelings and meanings in a way that really made sense to her. It felt *right* to her. Now if I try to access my own process of empathising, then it seems clear to me that although my mind wasn't lost in words and experiences my client had talked about several weeks before, my concentrated focus on her world as she experienced it clearly involved the specific area of my memory *as it pertained to that client*, and I could readily access this part of me. It feels a bit like being primed again – when I am with a particular client, I am primarily modulated to access memories *that relate to my knowledge of that client*. Of course I can access other memories if need be, yet they are maybe further removed from my immediate experiencing. So it feels as if when the client communicates to me, what I absorb 'floats around' in my knowing of that client, and sometimes connects with something that seems to have meaning *from within her own experience* that I have absorbed and retained. I realise that I am speaking off the cuff, but it feels as if *something* like that was going on within me.

As I was speaking, I was thinking ahead, too, and it occurs to me that my second example is different, and that feels good and interesting. It feels good because it illustrates diversity, and it interests me because this time the metaphor came from within me, not from my recall of the client's experience. This second client had been talking about how in some ways she resented her husband and felt disappointed because he didn't really understand her. She also spoke of how she didn't want to expose herself fully to him because he might feel hurt, so she was protecting his feelings. At one point (and I'm aware that this is only a small part of our total communication) I said something like:

> It feels a bit like a question in a maths paper – on the one hand you give him the numbers and the equals sign, but on the other hand you omit the plus, minus, multiply and divide signs because he might feel hurt by them. Then you feel disappointed when he doesn't come up with the right answer . . .

You know, as I said those words just then they sounded very judgemental! It really wasn't like that at all at the time, with the client. I'm feeling defensive! In context, my communication was fine, and the client responded with something along the lines of 'Wow! What a brilliant way of putting it! Yes, that's it *exactly*!'. And you know, I feel pretty confident that this enhanced awareness will make a real difference, if only at times, to the client's experiencing of herself and the way that she relates to her partner. Now if I think about what my processing was *at the time*, it feels as if I was again trying my hardest to absorb all that she was communicating, and again *what* I absorbed was 'floating around' my mind seeking some kind of referent. What emerged might have been from me, but it was very much related to trying to sense and feel how the client experienced herself and her relationship with her partner.

I've just remembered another example. I said to a client (I'll call her Jane for now) something like:

> It feels like you're in a tug of war with yourself. On one end of the rope there's all these big, hefty Janes and at the other end one tiny Jane. Yet somehow Baby Jane seems able to hold her ground.

This had real meaning for the client, and it seemed to really capture 'where she was at'. Anyway, yes, I think that when it seems to be an accurate way of communicating empathic understanding, I make use of metaphor and imagery quite a lot.

It occurs to me that the examples I have given don't quite do justice to the full process, as more often than not there is a *follow-up* to the use of metaphor. Even if, from the client's reaction, I am confident that I have accurately sensed the feeling, I need to determine whether ('perception check') I have also caught the meaning accurately, and vice versa. As with most if not all empathic communications, clients seem to take my words and then self-reference, and if we have established a therapeutic working alliance, they will feel free to come back with 'No, that's not quite it. . . . It's more like . . .'. Indeed, they may even choose to ignore my offering if it is not relevant or appropriate to them, in which case I believe that they nevertheless very much experience me as striving my hardest to sense how they experience themselves and their world, which is therapeutic in itself. Incidentally, I also believe that they feel safe and secure enough in our relationship to know that I will not take umbrage if they do ignore my metaphor.

In summary, I guess that the congruent and respectful use of metaphor (by which I mean that I am not simply using a technique, and am humble and tentative enough not to be adamant about appropriateness) is one of many effective ways of letting a client know that I really am committed to trying to empathically sense their feelings and meanings.

30 One last question? On the subject of being worn out, you spoke a while back about empathy being hard work. How do you avoid burnout?

Funnily enough, although I hear quite a few people talking about it, the prospect of 'burnout' is not something that bothers me personally. And you know, as I think about it, the people who talk about burnout tend to be teachers, lecturers, social workers, and so on – I don't recall too many *counsellors* talking about it. Maybe right now could be a good example. I've been talking for quite a while and I feel pretty tired, yet I also feel a sense of energy because I have enjoyed engaging with you, I have enjoyed and appreciated your engaging with me, and I also hope that I'll get some useful material out of this session! So I guess I'd say I'm something like 80% tired, fatigued or exhausted (because I've talked a lot and given out a lot) and 20% energised, invigorated or excited. When I have been with clients it usually feels different – perhaps nearer to fifty-fifty. There's something about being empathic (and congruent, and respectful) that is simultaneously draining but also edifying, or nourishing. It is draining because I put a great deal of effort into it. It is energising because it really is a privilege and honour to be allowed or welcomed into the private world of feelings and meanings of another person – I grow through this, too. So I experience both fatigue and exhilaration at one and the same time. It reminds me a little of what Rogers said about entropy and syntropy. Entropy is the ongoing decay of the universe, and there has been a long-held belief that ever since the Big Bang our universe has been dying. Yet ongoing trends towards growth, development and ever-increasing complexity have been acknowledged, too, and this is syntropy. So maybe the *effort* I put into empathising is like *entropy*, and the *privilege* and *personal growth* is like *syntropy*.

I thank you all.

Empathic understanding: in the necessary and sufficient conditions

For what we are about to receive

In Chapters 1, 2 and 3 we have to some degree looked at what empathic understanding is, in greater length have looked at what empathy is not, and have shared an interview about the process of empathising. Perhaps we can now place empathy back in the context of the necessary and sufficient conditions for therapeutic personality change as a whole.

Over the years, there has been much debate over just how many conditions there actually are – four, five, six, seven or eight. For instance, there would be only four conditions if conditions one and two (contact and client incongruence) were to be seen as *pre*-conditions, and only five conditions if condition one was regarded as a *pre*-condition. If either 'spirituality' or 'intuition' were to be seen as an additional condition, there would be seven in all, and if both were to be added, there would be eight. As Carl Rogers spoke of 'spirituality' (a term he viewed with some caution) as falling within conditions four and five and of 'intuition' as falling (mostly) within the realms of empathic understanding, these are not treated as separate or additional conditions in this book. Although there is truth in the statement that Carl Rogers sometimes wrote of condition one and sometimes of conditions one and two being *pre*-conditions in some senses, he nevertheless retained them within the entire version – likewise here.

Although there is, as we shall see, a logical rationale for the conditions appearing in the order that they do, it is worth remembering the rich interface between them. Just as Natalie Rogers was fearful of the essence of the I–thou relationship being lost through a nit-picking focus on minutiae, let us retain the essence of a client-centred relationship as a complex whole as we strive to place empathic understanding back within the context of this therapeutic interweave.

Empathy and contact

> I was trying to think about myself as a therapist in the therapeutic hour – as I seem to myself, and as I seem to be seen by others. I think one of the outstanding things is that I'm very much present to the client. I'm not sure entirely what I mean by that, but the main thing that's going on in me is my concern with, and attention to, and listening to the client. I'm very much present; nothing else matters much. That's why I can do a demonstration interview – it doesn't matter how many other people are around; for me there's just this one person that exists. What develops is a feeling of connectedness, and this is often very strongly felt by the client as well as by me, as though

> there is some kind of a real bond between us. That grows out of the fact
> that I do enter so fully into the client's personal world.
>
> (Rogers and Russell 2002: p. 280)

We shall now take a brief sidetrack of sorts. In his 1957 paper 'The necessary and
sufficient conditions of psychotherapeutic personality change' (Rogers 1957a),
Carl used the term *psychological contact*, and in his 1959 chapter 'A theory of
therapy, personality, and interpersonal relationships, as developed in the client-
centered framework' (Rogers 1959) he used the term *contact*. There has since been
much academic debate as to why the word 'psychological' was dropped. Well, it
wasn't. For the sake of historical accuracy if for no other reason, let it be known
that Carl Rogers wrote the 1959 chapter:

> much earlier than when it was published. I think it was written about
> 1953.
>
> (Frick 1989: p. 90)

So the 1959 version was penned *before* the 1957 paper. It was the slow process
between authorship and publication of a chapter in a *book* (to which other
psychologists were also contributing chapters) that meant that the 1959 version
appeared *after* the 1957 paper was presented and published in a *journal*. Thus the
debate about Carl 'dropping' the word 'psychological' makes no sense at all – the
more accurate detail is that he *added* the word! 'In which case', you might ask,
'why did Carl Rogers *add* the word "psychological" to his definition of two
persons being in contact?'. The answer is that no one really seems to know for
sure, although some speculate that it was because the 1957 paper was prepared
for the *Journal of Consulting Psychology*! The main reference used in this book is the
1959 version, which Carl himself said:

> was a very strenuous effort on my part to make some sense out of all
> my professional experience and personal experience up to that point.
>
> (Frick 1989: p. 90)

Although in the definitions that follow the use of the term 'psychological' would
seem, in context, to make sense, sometimes for the sake of brevity and to avoid
needless repetition only the word 'contact' is used. The meaning in each instance
remains the same.

Look – no couch!

The counselling process begins *before therapist and client actually meet*. In my own
practice, for instance, all would-be clients receive a leaflet that explains something
about me together with a basic overview of client-centred therapy. Rogers said:

> In the kind of therapeutic approach that makes sense to me, the more
> the individual knows of the climate I want to create, and of the
> principles that I believe to be operative, the more intelligently he
> can participate in the experience of therapy . . . For me, that is one
> reason for feeling that it is a more potent or widely useable theory: that
> it is not destroyed by people becoming aware of what is happening.
>
> (Rogers 1989: pp. 124–5)

Now imagine having a time machine and travelling back to the era when client-centred therapy was first being formulated. What might have been the norms at that time? Imagine that you arrive for your first appointment to be instructed by your analyst to lie:

> I've always found the notion of sitting behind a person who's lying on a couch and can't see [me] somewhat repugnant . . . I guess I felt this way because of many of the psychological connotations: I'm the expert; I'll observe what's going on in you, but I don't want to be present as a person; you adopt an unusual posture because this is now a very unusual situation, and it should produce all kinds of material you don't understand. All of that seemed a bit repugnant to me . . .
>
> (Rogers and Russell 2002: p. 246)

In client-centred therapy, however, even before the counsellor and the client meet, the therapist believes that:

> the opportunities for new learning are maximized when we approach the individual without a preconceived set of categories which we expect him to fit.
>
> (Rogers 1951: p. 497)

We probably take it pretty much for granted that we both sit, at even heights, face to face, yet this in itself is a statement about power sharing even as contact begins. Therapist values, attitudes and beliefs have great significance both *prior to* and at the *beginning* of a therapeutic relationship, for it:

> can be initiated by one party, without waiting for the other to be ready.
>
> (Rogers 1961: p. 336)

The therapist needs to be ready.

Look, listen and learn!

Sitting upright, face to face, at an even height communicates the therapist's respect for equality – the counsellor is not in sole control or in a superior position. This 'simple' or basic first impression gathers substance as the client-centred therapist refrains from taking a client case history, engaging in assessment or diagnostic procedures, or otherwise testing the client in some way. Nor is the therapist firing questions at the client. Rather, the client-centred therapist focuses their attention and their respectfully empathic capacities on striving to sense the client's world of feelings and meanings:

> Both client and therapist are implicitly directed to fix their attention on the client. This means that the therapist characteristically looks, listens, and otherwise attends to the client; the client characteristically looks into space or at some object in the room so as to focus on himself. The client, then, is in the spotlight, directed by the total situation and the power of the therapist's steady attentiveness to be conscious of himself. This kind of attention to the client and waiting for his initiative . . . energizes the situation, is an enormously powerful living out of the

belief in the organismic self, and casts the client steadily back on himself.

(Barton 1974: p. 186)

Thus statements such as 'This reminds me of' or 'It seems to me' or 'Have you considered . . .?' or 'I think that . . .' or 'This is clearly . . .' are not characteristic of client-centred therapy, in part because they shape the relationship around the therapist. Rather, the *client*-centred therapist *guards against* external intrusions into the client's world of feelings and meanings – the underlying message is that *you and only you matter to me.*

Relationship

In actual fact, Carl Rogers and his colleagues initially defined this first necessary and sufficient condition as neither 'contact' nor 'psychological contact' – the term used was *'relationship'*. However, this soon changed to 'two persons are in contact' due to the term *relationship* being experienced as too open to confusion and misunderstanding. For instance, some people seemed to interpret 'relationship' as meaning *deep* relationship, or *good* relationship, or *therapeutic* relationship, whereas:

The present term has been chosen to signify more clearly that this is the *least* or minimum experience which could be called a relationship.

(Rogers 1959: p. 207)

Carl Rogers never entirely abandoned the term *relationship*, though. In his later years, he often referred to Martin Buber and the notion of an 'I-thou' relation-ship:

When there is a real trendless immediacy in the relationship, when you're aware of nothing but this person and he's aware of nothing but you, and there is a deep sense of communication and unity between the two of you, that's the thing I refer to as I–Thou relationship.

(Rogers and Evans 1975: p. 25)

What, then, of such issues as age, gender, race, and social status? Rogers wrote that:

. . . it would appear that such elements as the sex, appearance, or mannerisms of the counselor play a lesser role than might be supposed. When the counselor is favorably perceived, it is as someone with warmth and interest for the client, someone with understanding.

(Rogers 1951: p. 69)

In effect, the therapist striving, and achieving to a significant degree, to be the 'core' client-centred conditions is more significant than social factors. When looking at empathy we saw that our own frames of reference contain within them counterparts to the perceptions of others, which enabled Carl to say:

As human beings trying to cope with life, to understand it and learn from it, we have vast pools of commonality to draw on. It makes no difference that I am an older white middle-class American male, and you may be yellow or black or communist or Israeli or Arab or Russian or young or female. If we are openly willing to share, then there is a large area in which understanding is possible.

> (Rogers 1978: p. 122)

Bearing in mind that the sixth necessary and sufficient condition is that the client perceives, *at least to a minimal degree*, the unconditional positive regard and empathic understanding of the therapist, it made sense to Rogers to define 'relationship' in *minimal* terms, thereby avoiding assumptions and value judgements about *good, deep*, and so on (and note, incidentally, the interconnection between conditions one and six). Returning to, clarifying and expanding on this, Carl wrote:

> This difference may be quite minimal and in fact not immediately apparent to an observer. Thus it might be difficult to know whether a catatonic patient perceives the therapist's presence as making a difference to him. But it is almost certain that at some physiological level he does sense or subceive this difference.
>
> (Rogers and Truax 1967: p. 99)

Two fundamental characteristics of relationship or (psychological) contact were deemed to be *safety* and (especially as the encounter progresses) *free communication*. How, then, might a safe and free relationship come about?

> And this basic security is not something the client believes because he is told, not something about which he convinces himself logically, it is something he experiences, with his own sensory and visceral equipment.
>
> (Rogers: 1951: p. 209)

Rogers wrote:

> We know that if the therapist holds within himself attitudes of deep respect and full acceptance for this client as he is, and similar attitudes toward the client's potentialities for dealing with himself and his situations; if these attitudes are suffused with a sufficient warmth, which transforms them into the most profound type of liking or affection for the core of the person; and if a level of communication is reached so that the client can begin to perceive that the therapist understands the feelings he is experiencing and accepts them at the full depth of that understanding, then we may be sure that the process is already initiated.
>
> (Rogers 1961: pp. 74–5)

Carl gave us several models of client-centred therapeutic process (*see* Chapter 5). In the 'seven-stage' version he stated that when in the first stage a client is unlikely to enter therapy, as there is a fixity and remoteness to the client's experiencing and an unwillingness to communicate the self (communicating instead only externalised feelings and meanings). In such a condition, clients do not embrace, recognise or own feelings and meanings due to their rigid self-concepts (rigid 'personal constructs' or 'configurations of self') and, as a defence, 'close and communicative relationships are construed as dangerous' and internal awareness is blocked. The client therefore does not experience in awareness any desire to change:

> In a deeply defended person . . . change is difficult to bring about. Change tends to occur more in the person who is already somewhat open-minded and searching in his approach to life.
>
> (Rogers and Evans 1975: p. 73)

(Again, then, we can see the potential in *open-minded seekers* prior to them even entering therapy.) For the deeply defended client, life tends to be perceived through the past rather than the present (so there is little or no 'immediacy'), and thinking is 'black and white' rather than gradational. Everything is everyone else's problem. It is unlikely that persons will either enter or benefit from therapy at this stage:

> We seem to know very little about how to provide the experience of being received for the person in the first stage, but it is occasionally achieved in play or group therapy where the person can be exposed to a receiving climate, without himself having to take any initiative, for a long enough time for him to experience himself *as received*.
>
> (Rogers 1961: p. 133)

Carl wondered, very tentatively, whether it might be more helpful to try to establish contact with very young clients, or 'extremely immature or regressed' people with conditional rather than unconditional positive regard:

> It seems clear that some immature or regressed clients may perceive a conditional caring as constituting more acceptance than an unconditional caring.
>
> (Rogers 1989: pp. 14–15)

Readers interested in stage-one characteristics might find some of the more recent work on pre-therapy helpful, such as *Pre-Therapy* by Garry Prouty, Dion van Werde and Marlis Portner (Prouty *et al.* 2002).

On several occasions Rogers pointed out that the condition that two persons are in contact could in fact be considered a *pre*-condition, for without this engagement in a relationship the predictions about establishing a therapeutic relationship that in turn would have predictable consequences in terms of personality change would be unlikely to follow. In terms of establishing whether or not contact exists:

> The simplest method of determination involves simply the awareness of both client and therapist. If each is aware of being in personal or psychological contact with the other, then this condition is met . . . The first condition of therapeutic change is such a simple one that perhaps it should be labeled an assumption or a precondition in order to set it apart from those that follow. Without it, however, the remaining items would have no meaning, and that is the reason for including it.
>
> (Rogers 1957a: pp. 95–103)

This could be restated using the *'If–then'* formula of client-centred theory, wherein necessary and sufficient condition one is the first 'if'. *If* two people make a perceived difference to one another, *then* the actualising of a potential becomes possible. (This formulaic version would continue 'and *if* one person is incongruent and *if* the other is congruently respectful and empathic, and *if* conditions four and five are perceived by the client in this relationship, *then* a client-centred therapeutic relationship ensues, and *if* this relationship exists, *then* predictable outcomes in client personality change occur'.) Carl Rogers wrote that only when clients experience themselves as fully *received* can they move on to stage two, wherein expression (albeit about non-self topics) begins to flow:

> I believe I can state this assumed condition in one word. . . . I shall assume that the client experiences himself as being fully *received*. By this I mean that whatever his feelings – fear, despair, insecurity, anger; whatever his mode of expression – silence, gestures, tears or words; whatever he finds himself being in this moment, he senses that he is psychologically *received*, just as he is, by the therapist. There is implied in this term the concept of being understood, empathically, and the concept of acceptance. It is also well to point out that it is the client's experience of this condition which makes it optimal, not merely the fact of its existence in the therapist.
>
> (Rogers 1961: pp. 130–31)

In stage two the client still externalises and feels little or no personal respons-ibility. Feelings may be exhibited but are disowned or are seen as past objects, rigid constructs are seen as facts, differentiation of feelings and meanings is limited or over-generalised; and, although contradictions may be expressed, they are not seen by the client as contradictions. If communication is not blocked – that is, if the client again feels fully *received* – then there is movement towards stage three. Having stated that one aspect of a client being received is free communication, Carl Rogers believed that a major factor in *impeding* interperso-nal communication 'is our very natural tendency to judge, to evaluate, to approve or disapprove . . .'. This tendency becomes more sharp or 'heightened' when feelings and emotions are deeply involved:

> So the stronger our feelings the more likely it is that there will be no mutual element in the communication. There will just be two ideas, two feelings, two judgments, missing each other in psychological space . . . This tendency to react to any emotionally meaningful statement by forming an evaluation of it from our own point of view is, I repeat, the major barrier to interpersonal communication.
>
> (Rogers 1961: pp. 331–4)

Here, then, is a direct link between *contact* (or *relationship*, or *receiving*) and *empathic understanding*, for Rogers gives us his solution to this major commun-ication barrier:

> Real communication occurs, and this evaluative tendency is avoided, when we listen with understanding.
>
> (Rogers 1961: pp. 331–4)

Although writing about group tensions at the time, there might nevertheless be a link with the client-centred therapist striving to receive clients fully and the place of supervision, personal therapy and peer networking, for Rogers stated that a *third party* can be of great help. If the third party is able to be non-evaluative and listen with understanding, like the supervisor clarifying the therapist's views and attitudes with an empathic acceptance, then the therapist will experience this acceptant understanding and be less prone to exaggeration, less defensive, less critical and more self-accepting. As a result the therapist is less inhibited about openly exploring how best to get as close as possible to being the therapist conditions.

The situational context is that clients arrive for therapy with an expectation that this wise healer will be of help. They feel distressed at what they perceive as their inability to cope with life. What have *clients* reported as being helpful in terms of the establishment of contact (or the beginning of a therapeutic relationship)? How might *clients* feel received? Rogers found that two words summarised this, namely *impersonal* and *secure*. How could a client-centred therapist be experienced as *impersonal*? Carl clarified as follows:

> This is obviously not intended to mean that the relationship was cold or disinterested. It appears to be the client's attempt to describe this unique experience in which the *person* of the counselor – the counselor as an evaluating, reacting person with needs of his own – is so clearly absent . . . the relationship is experienced as a one-way affair in a very unique sense. The whole relationship is composed of the self of the client, the counselor being depersonalized for purposes of therapy into being 'the client's other self'. It is this warm willingness on the part of the counselor to lay his own self temporarily aside, in order to enter into the experience of the client, which makes the relationship a completely unique one, unlike anything in the client's previous experience.
>
> (Rogers 1951: p. 208)

Clearly, in 1951 Carl took the view that therapist focus was entirely towards the client. While the construct of congruence developed over the years to include greater emphasis on therapist self-awareness too, Rogers never lost (as we shall see) his 'disciplined' attention to the client (usually to the extent of elimination of awareness of even an audience of hundreds).

Turning now to clients feeling safe and secure, Carl Rogers highlighted the importance of all three therapist conditions. With reference to *unconditional positive regard*, he maintained that a 'thoroughly consistent acceptance' was not at all linked with approval. Rather, it is an *absolute assurance* that the therapist will not evaluate, interpret, probe or foist personal opinion upon clients. As a consequence, clients feel less need to be defensive or to pretend anything in order to please their counsellor. Acceptance may be experienced by the client as supportive, yet it is not the therapist's intent to offer support. The therapist is alongside the client, not pushing from behind or towing – he or she is 'permitting' clients to choose any direction that they wish to take.

> The client does not feel that the therapist 'likes' him, in the usual sense of a biased and favourable judgment, and he is often not sure . . .

whether he likes the therapist . . . There is simply no evidence upon which such a judgment could be based. But that this is a secure experience, in which the self is deeply respected, that this is an experience in which there need be no fear of threat or attack – not even of the subtlest sort – of this the client gradually becomes sure.

> (Rogers 1951: pp. 208–9)

However, Carl linked client feelings of security in the therapeutic relationship with *empathy*, too:

> It is this which provides the ultimate in psychological safety, when added to the other two. If I say that I 'accept' you, but know nothing of you, this is a shallow acceptance indeed, and you realise that it may change if I actually come to know you. But if I understand you empathically, see you and what you are feeling and doing from your point of view, enter your private world and see it as it appears to you – and still accept you – then this is safety indeed. In this climate you can permit your real self to emerge, and to express itself in varied and novel formings as it relates to the world. This is a basic fostering of creativity.
>
> (Rogers 1951: p. 358)

Opening channels

Most clients *want* to enter therapy, although they would of course prefer not to be in a position where seeking therapy becomes necessary. When clients do feel in need of help, they go for it. In the context of education and student-centred learning, Rogers wrote:

> I think that you pick up a book or you go to a person because you want to learn something, which is quite different from teaching in the ordinary sense . . . teaching usually does mean the imparting of information, which is quite different from seeking what you want to learn . . . it is different from being visited by a seeker. . . . I can tell you it's a very different experience to be asked by a class to lecture on some given topic that they think I'm expert on, than it is to be pouring that same lecture on to them when they haven't asked for it. . . . I favor much more being visited by seekers than seeking to put something across.
>
> (Rogers 1989: p. 195)

The phrase 'you can read me like a book' comes to mind. In client-centred therapy, the client picks up their own book, and the book is them. The therapist is alongside clients as they compose, decompose and recompose themselves. Clients may well have been 'squashed by the system' and expect their counsellor to be the equivalent of a teacher, delivering didactic lectures and filling them full of knowledge. However, the therapist knows that the natural curiosity driven by their actualising tendency can be reawakened.

Perhaps the beginning of therapy could be characterised by the counsellor inviting the client to begin reading the book that is the client:

> *I have found it enriching to open channels whereby others can communicate their feelings, their private perceptual worlds, to me.* Because understanding is rewarding, I would like to reduce the barriers between others and me, so that they can, if they wish, reveal themselves more fully.
>
> ([Rogers 1961: p. 19)

Carl was keen to meet people as human beings *in a process of becoming*, rather than seeing people as bound up in the past (his or the client's) or through having his own aims to impose upon or guide the client's future. Perhaps the most extensive guidance with regard to the client-centred therapist establishing *contact* in a *relationship* in which the client feels *received* is to be found in the section entitled 'How can I create a helping relationship?' in *On Becoming A Person* (Rogers 1961: pp. 50–57). In these extracts, Carl Rogers offers ten questions that he had asked of himself when reflecting upon how he could be of most therapeutic help:

> a. Can I *be* in some way which will be perceived by the other person as trustworthy, as dependable or consistent in some deep sense?
>
> (Rogers 1961: p. 50)

In part this could be to do with aspects such as keeping appointments, being on time and respecting confidentiality. However, to *act* as consistent when inner experience is not in harmony with outer expression would, in the longer term, be perceived as inconsistent and untrustworthy. Thus Carl preferred to think in terms of being 'dependably real' rather than being 'rigidly consistent' (although once again it can be stressed that if inner experiencing is to match outer expression, the client-centred therapist will have conditions four and five – unconditional positive regard and empathic understanding – deeply integrated within this congruence). In summary, Carl said that when he was a unified and integrated person:

> I can *be* whatever I deeply *am*.
>
> (Rogers 1961: p. 51)

> b. Can I be expressive enough as a person that what I am will be communicated unambiguously?
>
> (Rogers 1961: p. 51)

In other words, *if* the therapist is in denial of (or is distorting to awareness) inner experiencing – that is, if the therapist is incongruent – *then* the client will perceive mixed or contradictory messages. This could be linked with the notion of reciprocal empathy. If the therapist's words are somehow out of synchronisation with paraverbal or non-verbal communicating, the client will sense this at some level.

> One way of putting this which may seem strange to you is that if I can form a helping relationship to myself – if I can be sensitively aware of and acceptant towards my own feelings – then the likelihood is great that I can form a helping relationship toward another.
>
> (Rogers 1961: p. 51)

Rogers believed that it is tremendously difficult to transparently be that which one is, and one consequence is that the facilitation of the growth of others through the therapist means that the therapist must grow, too. While this may be enriching, it is often also painful. Thus one characteristic that could be deemed necessary for the client-centred therapist is *courage*, for the therapist might fear being changed or influenced, or becoming lost in the world of the other. Carl believed the experience of client-centred therapy to be so wonderful, and yet quoted the possibility of personal change *for the therapist* as being a reason why it is not more widespread.

> c. Can I let myself experience positive attitudes toward this other person – attitudes of warmth, caring, liking, interest, respect?
>
> ([Rogers 1961: p. 52)

If I allow myself to freely experience such positive feelings toward another, might they somehow trap me? Might demands be made of me or might I be disappointed as an outcome of trusting? Carl Rogers believed that fears such as these are one explanation for a tendency to be 'professionally aloof' and to work in diagnostic, 'objective' ways. Yet:

> It is a real achievement when we can learn, even in certain relationships or at certain times in those relationships, that it is safe to care, that it is safe to relate to the other as a person for whom we have positive feelings.
>
> (Rogers 1961: p. 52)

> d. Can I be strong enough as a person to be separate from the other?
>
> (Rogers 1961: p. 52)

Carl stated that the therapist needs to be able to embrace *self*-respect as well as respect for clients, owning (and if needs be, communicating) personal feelings and meanings yet being clear that they belong to the therapist and not to the client. Is the therapist personally 'together' enough to be able to enter the world of client feelings and meanings without identifying with them, without drowning in or becoming depressed or engulfed by them? The therapist needs to be strong enough to really receive a client's anger or rage without being 'destroyed' by it, or to accept a client's feeling of love without becoming entrapped by that love, or somehow enslaved by it. When therapists experience and own their *personal power*, then they can engage with clients at deeper levels due to not being afraid of losing themselves.

> e. Am I secure enough within myself to permit him his separateness?
>
> (Rogers 1961: pp. 52–3)

Clearly linking with the last question, Rogers really needed to know whether he could permit people the *freedom to be* – and if therapists believe that clients should follow their advice or be dependent upon them, then clearly this is not so. He quoted a small, unpublished study conducted by Richard Farson, in which it was discovered that:

> The less well adjusted and less competent counselor tends to induce conformity to himself, to have clients who model themselves after him.
>
> (Farson 1955)

However, better-adjusted (that is, more congruent) counsellors do not interfere with the freedom of clients to be themselves.

> f. Can I let myself enter fully into the world of his feelings and personal meanings and see these as he does?
>
> (Rogers 1961: p. 53)

Carl Rogers experienced an immersion in the world of clients so deep that all desire to evaluate or judge them dissipated. Sensitive and accurate empathic understanding is not just of the obvious, but also of implicit, dimly perceived and confused meanings, and on an ongoing basis.

> g. Can I receive him as he is? Can I communicate this attitude? Or can I only receive . . . conditionally?
>
> (Rogers 1961: p. 54)

Disapproval of some feelings, whether openly or silently, is not a hallmark of client-centred therapy. Ideally, the therapist is open to and accepting of each and every facet or aspect that the client chooses to be in therapy. Carl Rogers, if he experienced evaluative feelings, would explore where they might have come from:

> And when – afterward and sometimes too late – I try to discover why I have been unable to accept him in every respect, I usually discover that it is because I have been frightened or threatened in myself by some aspect of his feelings. If I am to be more helpful, then I must myself grow and accept myself in these respects.
>
> (Rogers 1961: p. 54)

We see once again, then, the value of personal growth activities for the therapist (or trainee therapist), the value of good, person-centred supervision, and the value of networking with like-minded peers.

> h. Can I act with sufficient sensitivity in the relationship that my behavior will not be perceived as a threat?
>
> (Rogers 1961, p. 54)

Rogers explained that this was not about being hypersensitive to clients, although physiological research evidence indicates that even communicating a word only slightly stronger in meaning than that which the client used does produce a threat reaction. Rather:

> It is simply due to the conviction based on experience that if I can free him as completely as possible from external threat, then he can begin to experience and to deal with the internal feelings and conflicts which he finds threatening within himself.
>
> (Rogers 1961: p. 54)

> i. Can I free him from the threat of external evaluation
>
> (Rogers 1961: p. 54)

Related to the previous question, this one is specifically to do with the punishment and reward systems that nearly all (if not all) people meet with from birth to death – *good* or *bad*, *pass* or *fail*, *worthy* or *shameful*, and so on. Rogers believed that such evaluations are not at all facilitative of personal growth and therefore play no part in a client-centred therapeutic relationship – and this includes positive judgements, for as we have already seen, the right to praise (to cite just one example) implies the right to chastise or withhold praise.

> So I have come to feel that the more I can keep a relationship free of judgment and evaluation, the more this will permit the other person to reach the point where he recognizes that the locus of evaluation, the center of responsibility, lies within himself.
>
> (Rogers 1961: p. 55)

The client-centred therapist strives to reach a state of congruence wherein there is no inner evaluation of clients, let alone communicated judgements. Ideally, there is not even any *desire* to be evaluative – the optimum desire is to authentically and respectfully understand.

> j. Can I meet this other individual as a person who is in a process of *becoming*, or will I be bound by his past and my past?
>
> (Rogers 1961: p. 55)

Any preconceived ideas or notions that the therapist holds about a client serve to limit what that client can be in the therapeutic relationship. Rogers quoted Martin Buber, who wrote about *confirming the other:*

> Confirming means . . . accepting the whole potentiality of the other . . . I can recognize in him, know in him, the person he has been . . . *created* to become . . . I can confirm him in myself, and then in him, in relation to this potentiality that . . . can now be developed, can evolve.
>
> (Rogers and Buber 1957)

As Carl stated, if the client is perceived as someone already bound by the past, already categorised and fixed in time, this is very, very different from receiving a person who is in a *process of becoming*.

In summary, Carl Rogers wrote of his exploration of personal characteristics relevant to entering or initiating therapeutic contact:

> . . . the optimal helping relationship is the kind of relationship created by a person who is psychologically mature. Or to put it another way, the degree to which I can create relationships which facilitate the growth of others as separate persons is a measure of the growth I have achieved in myself. In some respects this is a disturbing thought, but it is also a promising or challenging one. It would indicate that if I am interested in creating helping relationships, I have a fascinating lifetime job ahead of me, stretching and developing my potentialities in the direction of growth.
>
> (Rogers 1961: p. 56)

Contact – chocks away!

It is perhaps to be regretted that almost inevitably the six necessary and sufficient conditions for therapeutic personality change are represented as a vertical yet linear hierarchy – a *top-to-bottom* list with each aspect following the one above it.

Although there is a rationale for certain conditions preceding others (for instance, without relationship there is no process or outcomes, and unconditional positive regard and empathic understanding need to be perceived as authentic), when placing empathy back in the context of all six necessary and sufficient conditions, it will become evident that all six conditions interweave, very much relating to and being integrated with one another. A slightly less linear diagrammatic representation might be that within the context of two individuals who are in psychological contact.

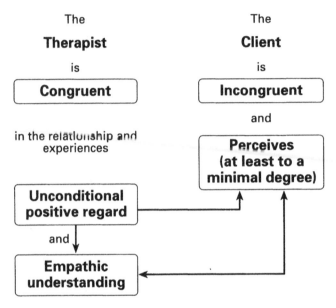

Figure 4.1 An illustration of the interface between counsellor and client in the process of client-centred therapy.

Thus the counsellor is congruent in this therapeutic relationship. Integral to this congruence is the experiencing of unconditional positive regard towards and empathic understanding of an incongruent client, who perceives this empathic understanding (at least to a minimal degree, and in part through a process of reciprocal empathy) and, via that understanding, the unconditional positive regard of the therapist.

Experience will be defined (in different ways) shortly. As Rogers wrote of *contact* meaning that the therapist and client 'each make a perceived or subceived difference in the experiential field of the other', it might be helpful to explore briefly the meaning of some of the terms used. We can begin with *'each makes a perceived . . .'*.

Carl Rogers (and others, such as Hebb and Riesen) believed that the 'impingement of stimuli' and the 'meaning given to the stimuli' are 'inseparable parts of a single experience' (that is, the instant we *experience* something we attach a *meaning* to it):

> perception is a hypothesis or prognosis for action which comes into being in awareness when stimuli impinge on the organism. When we perceive 'this is a triangle', 'that is a tree', 'this person is my mother', it

means that we are making a prediction that the objects from which the stimuli are received would, if checked in other ways, exhibit properties we have come to regard, from our past experience, as being character-istic of triangles, trees, mother.

(Rogers 1959: p. 199)

Thus Carl reckoned that the terms *perception* and *awareness* were more or less synonymous, although he tended to use the term *perception* in the more detailed sense that emphasised the stimulus (that which is being perceived), whereas *awareness* included the symbolisations and meanings associated with that which is being perceived, as well as memory traces and physiological changes connected to the perception.

With regard to the meaning of *'each makes a perceived or subceived . . .'*, Rogers drew on the work of McCleary and Lazarus, who stated that:

even when a subject is unable to report a visual discrimination he is still able to make a stimulus discrimination at some level below that required for conscious recognition.

(McCleary and Lazarus 1949: pp. 171–9)

Carl incorporated the process of discrimination without awareness, known as *subception*, into client-centred personality theory, stating that:

It is this capacity which, in our theory, permits the individual to discriminate an experience as threatening, without symbolization in awareness of this threat.

(Rogers 1959: p. 200)

One of the capacities of human beings that distinguishes us from many other animals is that we do have a significant capacity for awareness:

We have a rich capacity for symbolization, which I believe is synon-ymous with awareness. We have the capacity for a rich subjective living. We have the capacity for an organismic valuing process. That is, we are able to test objects and events in terms of our own experiencing and can gauge the values they have for enhancing us or for being destructive in our experience.

(Rogers 1989: p. 120)

Carl Rogers saw *symbolisation* and *awareness* (and indeed *consciousness*) as meaning essentially the same thing:

consciousness (or awareness) is the symbolization of some of our experience. Awareness is thus seen as the symbolic representation (not necessarily in verbal symbols) of some portion of our experience. This representation may have varying degrees of sharpness or vivid-ness, from a dim awareness of something existing as ground, to a sharp awareness of something which is in focus as figure.

(Rogers 1959: p. 198)

When asked by Richard Evans whether his own view of consciousness paralleled the theory promulgated by Sigmund Freud, Carl Rogers replied:

> I feel that whether or not I totally agree or disagree (with Freud's concept of the unconscious) is, in itself, not very helpful. I'd rather point out the way I conceptualize . . .
>
> (Rogers and Evans 1975: p. 7)

And Carl did point out the way he thought of awareness when he said:

> I'd prefer to think of a range of phenomena: first, those in sharp focus in awareness right now – the height of consciousness; secondly, a range of material which could be called into consciousness, that you really know and can call into consciousness but you don't have in 'figure' right now – it is in the 'ground' or background; then, finally, some phenomena which are more and more dimly connected with awareness, to material that is really prevented from coming into even vague awareness because its coming into awareness would damage the person's concept of himself.
>
> (Rogers and Evans 1975: p. 6)

When there is an absence of psychological defensive processes, experience can be symbolised freely and is hence deemed to be *available to awareness*. In defining *accurate symbolisation*, Rogers wrote:

> The symbols which constitute our awareness do not necessarily match, or correspond to, the 'real' experience, or to 'reality'. Thus the psychotic is aware of (symbolizes) electrical impulses in his body which do not seem in actuality to exist. I glance up quickly and perceive a plane in the distance, but it turns out to be a gnat close to my eye. It seems important to distinguish between those awarenesses which, in common-sense terms, are real or accurate and those which are not.
>
> (Rogers 1959: p. 198)

Stating that the examples given above are, effectively, *perceptual hypotheses* that can be checked (for instance, by brushing at the speck it might become more clear that it was a gnat and not an aeroplane), and while acknowledging this link between symbolisation and perception, Rogers nevertheless was able to state that:

> when we speak of accurate symbolization in awareness, we mean that the hypotheses implicit in the awareness will be borne out if tested by acting on them.
>
> (Rogers 1959: p. 199)

The notion of two people being in contact will be examined again when we look at the sixth necessary and sufficient condition (the client *perceiving*, at least to a minimal degree, the fourth and fifth conditions, namely the *unconditional positive regard* of the therapist, and the *empathic understanding* of the therapist). For the moment, let us note a subtle yet significant difference. Person A (who is relatively incongruent) and person B (who is relatively congruent) are in contact. However, person A is unable or unwilling (for whatever reason) to *perceive* (even to a minimal degree) the authentic unconditional positive regard and empathic understanding of person B. In this scenario, it is far less likely that a therapeutic relationship will be a consequence of their contact.

As we relocate empathic understanding within all six necessary and sufficient conditions, let us also note, in summary, that integral to the nature of this *contact*, this *psychological contact*, this *relationship* between two people, is the commitment of the therapist to experience genuine respect and empathy for and of the client's world of feelings and personal meanings.

Empathy and client incongruence

One meaning of congruence and incongruence relates to geometric shapes. If two shapes can be exactly superimposed they are said to be *congruent*; if they do not exactly fit over one another and match, they are said to be *incongruent*.

Carl Rogers believed that the human organism has one, and only one, basic motivation – to maintain and enhance itself. This 'function' is 'undertaken' by the *actualising tendency*:

> This is the inherent tendency of the organism to develop all its capacities in ways which serve to maintain or enhance the organism. . . . It should also be noted that it is the organism as a whole, and only the organism as a whole, which exhibits this tendency . . . The self, for example, is an important construct in our theory, but the self does not 'do' anything. It is only one expression of the general tendency of the organism to behave in those ways which maintain and enhance itself. . . . It might also be mentioned that such concepts of motivation as are termed need-reduction, tension-reduction, drive-reduction, are included in this concept. It also includes, however, the growth motivations which appear to go beyond these terms: the seeking of pleasurable tensions, the tendency to be creative, the tendency to learn painfully to walk when crawling would meet the same needs more comfortably.
>
> (Rogers 1959: p. 196)

Carl Rogers and human nature

What it means to be a human being is of central significance in client-centred theory. When asked about where he would place himself in a continuum stretching from humanistic to psychoanalytic and behavioural, Rogers said of psychoanalytic thinking and practice:

> I think that it really is a damaging cultural influence, as it gets spread more widely in an oversimplified form. I think Freud's view that man is by nature evil and that the id is a terrible force which, if released, would play havoc, could lead to damage.
>
> (Rogers and Evans 1975: p. 71)

In response to where Rogers would locate himself, his view was that:

> there is a flavor of existentialism developing which is definitely positive in its view of man, and I certainly would have to place myself there.
>
> (Rogers and Evans 1975: p. 71)

Carl Rogers would not say, though, that he was a 'pure' existentialist because he thought that:

> some of the existentialists take the point of view that man really has no nature, but it seems to me that he has – I have taken the point of view that man belongs to a particular species. He has species characteristics. One of those, I think, being the fact that he is incurably social; I think he has a deep need for relationships. Then I think that simply because man is an organism he tends to be directional. He's moving in the direction of actualizing himself. So, for myself, I really feel man does have a describable nature.
>
> (Rogers 1989: p. 66)

Returning to the theme of psychoanalysis, Carl Rogers despised the view that at the 'heart' of human beings lie instincts and impulses that must be controlled, because his own experience led him to believe that:

> if we can release what is most basic in the individual, it will be constructive . . . when you get to what is deepest in the individual, that is the very aspect that can be most trusted to be constructive or to tend toward socialization or toward the development of better interpersonal relationships.
>
> (Rogers 1989: p. 58)

He stated many times that of course 'negative' feelings will be disclosed in psychotherapy, and that each and every one of us has the capacity for 'evil' behaviour. However:

> It is well to bear in mind that I also have a capacity to vomit, for example. Whether I, or anyone, will translate the impulses into behavior depends, it seems to me, on two elements: social conditioning and voluntary choice.
>
> (Rogers 1989: p. 254)

So the fact that we all have the *potential* to behave in antisocial ways does not have to mean that such ways are our base nature. On the contrary:

> I find in my experience no . . . innate tendency toward destructiveness, toward evil . . . if the elements making for growth are present, the actualizing tendency develops in positive ways. In the human these elements for growth are not only proper nutrition etc., but a climate of psychological attitudes.
>
> (Rogers 1989: pp. 253–4)

In terms of the 'nature versus nurture' debate, Rogers said that:

> I see members of the human species . . . as *essentially* constructive in their fundamental nature, but damaged by their experience.
>
> (Rogers 1981: p. 238)

Some years later:

> Viewed from the external, scientific, objective perspective, man is determined by genetic and cultural influences. I have also said that

in an entirely different dimension, such things as freedom and choice are extremely real.

(Rogers 1989: p. 132)

Growth is not a balancing act!

Very often, mental health is seen as trying to achieve *balance*. Yet the actualising tendency is *not* seeking balance – far from it. Balance in this sense would stem, thwart or stifle evolution and growth:

> I think the organism is definitely not trying to achieve *stasis*. I think that even organisms as low as the flatworm are always trying to look for more enriching stimuli, more complicated stimuli . . .
>
> (Rogers and Evans 1975: p. 3)

Richard Evans queried whether Carl meant that actually at some deep level human beings seek rather than strive to avoid tensions. Rogers replied:

> Always. I think there is plenty of evidence now that this is true. In man, we call it curiosity.
>
> (Rogers and Evans 1975: p. 3)

It was fundamental to Carl's belief system that the central motivating aspect of every person is a tendency toward *maintaining* the entire organism and, whenever possible, *enhancing* the organism, too – and given the right conditions, growth will be in a constructive not a destructive direction:

> I've said sometimes that my generally optimistic point of view could be glandular; I don't know. One facet of this is certainly true – there's no doubt that my interest in growth is positive.
>
> (Rogers and Evans 1975: p. 71)

The self

As a human being grows, a *portion* of the whole organism (and both Carl Rogers and Sigmund Freud were in agreement that this was a relatively small fraction of the whole) becomes *differentiated* as the *self*. The actualising tendency now 'gets to work' on the self, or self-concept – so the *self* now strives to maintain and enhance itself, often at the expense of the organism as a whole.

> Following the development of the self-structure, this general tendency toward actualization expresses itself also in the actualization of that portion of the experience of the organism which is symbolized in the self. If the self and the total experience of the organism are relatively congruent, then the actualizing tendency remains relatively unified. If self and experience are incongruent, then the general tendency to actualize the organism may work at cross purposes with the subsystem of that motive, the tendency to actualize the self.
>
> (Rogers 1959: pp. 196–7)

I confess to 'having an agenda' here, for it alarms me that so many practitioners who undertook client-centred training seem unaware of the fundamental distinction between the actualising tendency and self-actualising. Imagine, if you will, the self being akin to a small yolk in a large egg. The egg is the entire organism, and the yolk is but a differentiated part. The actualising tendency is a motivational force for the whole egg, self-actualising for the yolk only (examples to illustrate this follow soon).

Going back to geometric shapes, incongruence means that there is a mismatch between one shape, the entire human organism, and the other shape, that portion of the whole organism that has become differentiated as the self. Another way of illustrating this might be to see the two shapes as *experience* and our *perception* of that experience. If our perception of our experiencing is at odds with organismic experiencing (that is, experiencing by the total organism and not just the differentiated part of it known as the self), we are in a state of incongruence.

When exploring and defining *experience*, Carl Rogers differentiated between *experience as a noun, experience as a verb*, and *experiencing a feeling. Experience* as a *noun* means:

> all that is going on within the envelope of the organism at any given moment which is potentially available to awareness. It includes events of which the individual is unaware, as well as all the phenomena which are in consciousness. Thus it includes the psychological aspects of hunger, even though the individual may be so fascinated by his work or play that he is completely unaware of the hunger; it includes the impact of sights and sounds and smells on the organism, even though these are not in the focus of attention. It includes the influence of memory and past experience, as these are active in the moment, in restricting or broadening the meaning given to various stimuli. It also includes all that is present in immediate awareness or consciousness. It does not include such events as neuron discharges or changes in blood sugar, because these are not directly available to awareness. It is thus a psychological, not a physiological definition.
>
> (Rogers 1959: p. 197)

Stating that in the past he had used phrases for experience (as a *noun*) like *organismic experiencing* and *sensory and visceral experiences* (the viscera are the large cavities and organs in the body), Rogers stated that other synonyms included *experiential field* or *phenomenal field*. It was the *'totality'* of the concept of experiencing that he wished to convey – that experience means more than simply *conscious* experiencing. He also clarified that experience in this sense refers to *here and now* experience rather than an accumulation of historic experiencing. Thus as a *noun*, experience refers to *an* experience.

Experience as a *verb* means simply that sensory or physiological events happening in the moment are received (or impact upon) the organism. Again Rogers clarified:

> Often this process term is used in the phrase 'to experience in awareness', which means to symbolize in some accurate form at the conscious level the above sensory or visceral events. Since there are varying degrees of completeness in symbolization, the phrase is often 'to experience more fully in awareness', thus indicating that it is the

extension of this process toward more complete and accurate symbolization to which reference is being made.

(Rogers 1959: pp. 197–8)

In other words, experiencing may be denied symbolisation in awareness altogether. However, if experiencing is granted conscious recognition yet only in a distorted fashion, there are clearly *degrees* of distortion. Another way of putting this is to consider that rather than an individual either being totally aware or totally unaware, there is a continuum between these two extremes, different degrees of conscious awareness (again, examples follow shortly). Finally, there is Carl's definition of *experiencing a feeling*:

> This is a term which has been heavily used in writings on client-centered therapy and theory. It denotes an emotionally tinged experience, together with its personal meaning. Thus it includes the emotion but also the cognitive content of the meaning of that emotion in its experiential context. It thus refers to the unity of emotion and cognition as they are experienced inseparably in the moment. It is perhaps best thought of as a brief theme of experience, carrying with it the emotional coloring and the perceived meaning to the individual. Examples would include 'I feel angry at myself', 'I feel ashamed of my desires when I am with her', 'For the first time, right now, I feel that you like me'. This last is an example of another phenomenon which is relevant to our theory, and which has been called *experiencing a feeling fully*, in the immediate present.
>
> (Rogers 1959: p. 198)

Where does all of this *experiencing* take place, especially experiencing that the individual is aware or conscious of (experience that is symbolised)? Originally, Carl Rogers was not particularly interested in a concept as 'woolly' or meaningless or ambiguous as the *self*. However, as client after client after client kept referring to being aware of experience and meanings in this thing they called a 'self', he eventually thought that to honour them he had best acknowledge it in some way:

> I think I'll talk a little bit about the concept of *self*, because that's a very central aspect of my theory. It seemed to me that self could be defined in many, many different ways, and many of them acceptable, but what definition would be most profitable for consideration in research and in thinking? It seemed to me that the most useful definition was that the self was composed of the perceptions that the individual had of the 'I' or the 'me', the perceptions of the self in relationship to others and to the environment, and the values that were attached to those perceptions. So it was a definition which was all based on perceptions by the individual, and those could be determined – could conceivably be measured, though for a long time I didn't see how they could be measured.
>
> (Rogers and Russell 2002: pp. 247–8)

Rogers also said that although social conditioning was undoubtedly a factor in the building of a self, the self was more fluid than a fixed, built construction. He came to this conclusion in part through his experiencing of clients and in part through being a client himself. On being a client, Rogers said:

> I could go away from an interview feeling, 'I really am a worthwhile person; I do like myself; I'm okay'; but then some little incident could flip that feeling over while it was still tentative and newborn, and I would feel, 'I'm really no good; I'm a fraud; I'm not much good'. It was quite fascinating to me – not very comfortable, but fascinating – to look back a little bit and see how, in a moment of time, that whole gestalt could shift. And that happened in my clients, too. Very definitely.
>
> (Rogers and Russell 2002: pp. 247–8)

Unlike many other psychologists, however, Rogers opted not to tread the path of trying to predict or determine physical brain structures (for instance, Freud believed that it was only a matter of time before the physical locations of the id, ego and superego would be found in the human brain), or to relate human psychological development to specific phases or ages (such as Freud's psychosexual theories or Piaget's 'life span' stages). Nor was Rogers overly engaged with colleagues and students working on the notion of different selves, and configurations of self:

> It should be mentioned that some students of mine stressed too much, perhaps, the notion of different selves, although I don't quarrel with that idea particularly. This idea hasn't had as much meaning for me as the notion of a more complex unified picture of self which keeps expanding to include new experiences, even though some experiences may be shut out as being too threatening. It seems that each of us endeavors to preserve the concept or picture that he has of himself and that a sharp change in that picture is quite threatening. Any change destroys some of the security that we feel we need.
>
> (Rogers and Evans 1975: p. 17)

It might be that evidence from neuroscience comes close to corroborating Carl's notion of a shifting or fluid self. Professor Susan Greenfield wrote:

> There is no 'centre' for consciousness – after all, that would mean we have a complete mini-brain in a brain.
>
> (Greenfield 2000: p. 176)

Likewise, there is no single centre (or 'mini-brain') for unconsciousness, or for being non-conscious. With regard to a sense of self, Greenfield thinks in terms of what she calls a *transient self* – in other words, the kind of fluid self that Carl Rogers wrote and spoke of. According to Greenfield:

> At some global level of organization, then, beyond a single cell and beyond any rigidly demarcated edifice in the brain, we might imagine an assembly of neurons so large that it does not respect any particular anatomical boundary, and at the same time one that is fast and evanescent enough to permit the formation of another, different and dominant assembly a moment later.
>
> (Greenfield 2000: p. 176)

It could just be, then, that a personal construct (George Kelly) or a configuration of self (Rogers, then Mearns) is analogous to an assembly of neurons that at any given time can become dominant. At the same time, the sense of self might be transient, a constant and complex flow within the brain. Perhaps the notion of rigidity of constructs could be linked with the notion that:

> Connectivity between and among assemblies of neurons creates in advance a dominant assembly that prevents competing assemblies from forming.
>
> (Greenfield 2000: p. 181)

Incidentally, such neuroscientific thinking might also be linked with Carl's notion of the client-centred therapist being disciplined and the idea of the therapist being modulated for receiving clients empathically. Of modulation:

> We know that neurotransmitters can say more than just yes or no – they can 'modulate' a target cell, not giving a signal directly but, more subtly, putting the cell on red alert.
>
> (Greenfield 2000: p. 100)

Furthermore, it may even be possible that unless cells have a modulated status, they may not react at all, and:

> when we speak of modulation, it is always with reference to two events occurring one after the other within a limited timeframe.
>
> (Greenfield 2000: p. 100)

Might this relate to a client disclosing, followed by the therapist's perception of that disclosure, followed by the therapist's attempt to understand that disclosure, followed by the therapist communicating the outcome of this process?

Anyway, Carl Rogers thought very much in terms of an *ongoing process of becoming a person*, yet this did not prevent the research and development of a client-centred theory of personality.

Having explored the notion of a self, we can now turn to definitions of *self-experience, self, concept of self* and *self-structure*. *Self-experience* was considered to be the raw data out of which the concept of self is formed and organised. In defining *self, concept of self* and *self-structure*, Rogers wrote:

> These terms refer to the organized, consistent, conceptual gestalt composed of perceptions of the characteristics of the 'I' or 'me' and the perceptions of the relationships of the 'I' or 'me' to others and to various aspects of life, together with the values attached to these perceptions. It is a gestalt which is available to awareness though not necessarily in awareness. It is a fluid and changing gestalt, a process, but at any given moment it is a specific entity which is at least partially definable in operational terms . . . The term self or self-concept is more likely to be used when we are talking of the person's view of himself, self-structure when we are looking at this gestalt from an external frame of reference.
>
> (Rogers 1959: p. 200)

Carl Rogers also wrote of the *ideal self*, which denotes the self-concept that is valued most highly and that a person would most like to have.

So the human infant is born with an *actualising tendency*, a motivational force akin to the inherent potential of an acorn to become a flourishing oak tree (and an acorn *does* strive to become a flourishing oak tree – and *given the right conditions, it will* become all that it can be). This actualising tendency is constructive and tends towards growth and complexity. As Carl wrote, we are less likely to actualise our potential for migraine than our potential for tasty food. Thus the actualising tendency, striving to maintain and enhance the whole human organism, is positive and trustworthy in nature. However, a portion of the whole organism becomes differentiated, *through interaction with the environment,* as the self. This led Rogers and his colleagues to think about how this self might develop and be constructed, and a key emergent idea was the notion of a *regard complex*:

> The regard complex is a construct defined by Standal as all those self-experiences, together with their interrelationships, which the individual discriminates as being related to the positive regard of a particular social other.
>
> This construct is intended to emphasize the gestalt nature of transactions involving positive or negative regard, and their potency. Thus, for example, if a parent shows positive regard to a child in relationship to a specific behavior, this tends to strengthen the whole pattern of positive regard which has previously been experienced as coming from that parent. Likewise specific negative regard from this parent tends to weaken the whole configuration of positive regard.
>
> (Rogers 1959: pp. 208–9)

As the self is becoming differentiated from the organism as a whole, certain human needs become evident. The *need for positive regard* is a need to feel liked, loved, valued, appreciated, and considered as being of worth, especially by 'significant others' (such as close family or carers initially, and later by friends, teachers, and so on). First we shall consider the meaning of *positive regard*, then the *need for positive regard*:

> In general, positive regard is defined as including such attitudes as warmth, liking, respect, sympathy, acceptance. To perceive oneself as receiving positive regard is to experience oneself as making a positive difference in the experiential field of another.
>
> It is postulated by Standal that a basic need for positive regard, as defined above, is a secondary or learned need, commonly developed in early infancy. Some writers have looked upon the infant's need for love and affection as an inherent or instinctive need. Standal is probably on safer ground in regarding it as a learned need. By terming it the need for positive regard, he has, it is believed, selected out the significant psychological variable from the broader terms usually used.
>
> (Rogers 1959: p. 208)

Client-centred theorists believe that most human relationships are *conditional*. Conditional relationships involve values and judgements, as in *'I like you when . . .',*

'I love you when . . .', *'I value you most when . . .'*, *'I really appreciate it when you . . .'*, and so on. The reverse, of course, is also true: *'I don't like it when you . . .'*, *'I hate it when you . . .'*, and so on. Now due to the desire (or need) for positive regard from significant others, the young human being quickly learns that it is usually best to adapt to the values and judgements of others, to behave in ways that are more likely to result in positive, not negative, regard – better to be loved than to be hated . . .

Another development is the *need for positive self-regard*:

> This term is used to denote a positive regard satisfaction which has become associated with a particular self-experience or a group of self-experiences, in which this satisfaction is independent of positive regard transactions with social others. Though it appears that positive regard must first be experienced from others, this results in a positive attitude toward self which is no longer directly dependent on the attitudes of others. The individual, in effect, becomes his own significant social other.
>
> (Rogers 1959: p. 209)

In other words, we value *ourselves* via the values that we have taken on (or 'introjected') from *others*. Thus the young girl might learn that *caring* for dolls and *pleasing others* is very acceptable to a parent, as is *being seen but not heard*. Due to this child's need to feel liked and loved by and acceptable to that parent, she mostly behaves in a way that elicits responses from the parent that feel internally pleasurable, rather than risking the likelihood of unpleasant internal feelings that are a consequence of parental disapproval. However, if 'being seen but not heard' is internalised (or introjected) by this young girl as a 'good' value – albeit based on the evaluative attitudes of a parent and not on her own, direct, organismic valuing – then she may come to value herself for being seen and not heard even when the relevant parent is not around. Consider another example. How often do we (in the UK, at least) come across the perception that men are less adept than women at expressing their feelings? The answer is very often. Does the aphorism 'big boys don't cry' also 'ring a bell'? Suppose that a young boy injures himself while playing, and hears a significant adult remark 'big boys don't cry'. Needing to be valued, the boy therefore doesn't weep. This value may then be introjected *as if* it were direct organismic valuing, so that the next time he suffers an injury while playing, the boy feels good about himself for holding back his tears even though there are no significant adults around. He thus satisfies his need for positive *self*-regard. The *organismic* experience (based on an *internal locus of evaluation*) of the young girl is that sometimes it feels good to smash up a doll and scream. The *organismic* valuing (again based on an *internal locus of evaluation*) of the boy is that sometimes it feels good to sob and get cuddled. In both instances, however, their *perceptions* of their experiencing come to include *introjected values*, and organismic valuing is therefore denied or distorted. The individual still experiences a positive feeling about *self* through feeling that they have lived up to their introjected values – values that have effectively become *independent* of significant others (in effect, the individual has become his or her own significant other).

Two further dimensions complete the gestalt of an individual's regard complex:

Need for self-regard. It is postulated that a need for positive self-regard is a secondary or learned need, related to the satisfaction of the need for positive regard by others.

Unconditional self-regard. When the individual perceives himself in such a way that no self-experience can be discriminated as more or less worthy of positive regard than any other, then he is experiencing unconditional positive self-regard.

(Rogers 1959: p. 209)

Other definitions relevant to the preceding scenario are of *locus of evaluation* and *organismic valuing*. We shall begin with *locus of evaluation*:

This term is used to indicate the source of evidence as to values. Thus an internal locus of evaluation, within the individual himself, means that he is the center of the valuing process, the evidence being supplied by his own senses. When the locus of evaluation resides in others, their judgment as to the value of an object or experience becomes the criterion of value for the individual.

(Rogers 1959: p. 210)

Organismic valuing refers to:

an ongoing process in which values are never fixed or rigid, but experiences are being accurately symbolized and continually and freshly valued in terms of the satisfactions organismically experienced; the organism experiences satisfaction in those stimuli or behaviors which maintain and enhance the organism and the self, both in the immediate present and in the long range. The actualizing tendency is thus the criterion. The simplest example is the infant who at one moment values food, and when satiated, is disgusted with it; at one moment values stimulation, and soon after, values only rest; who finds satisfying that diet which in the long run most enhances his development.

(Rogers 1959: p. 210)

We have learned, though, that *self-actualising* (maintaining and enhancing the *self-concept*, formulated around our *conditions of worth*) – despite feeling good within the self – can nevertheless serve to *thwart* the *actualising tendency* (based on *organismic valuing processes*). In such instances, the individual is in a state of *incongruence*:

It seems to me that the infant is not estranged from himself. To me it seems that the infant is a whole and integrated organism, gradually individual, and that the estrangement that occurs is one that he learns – that in order to preserve the love of others, parents usually, he takes into himself as something he has experienced for himself, the judgments of his parents: just like the small boy who has been rebuked for pulling his sister's hair goes around saying, 'bad boy, bad boy'. Meanwhile, he is pulling her hair again. In other words, he has introjected the notion that he is bad, where actually he is enjoying the experience, and it is this estrangement between what he is experiencing and the concepts he links up with what he is experiencing that seems to me to constitute the basic estrangement.

(Rogers 1989: p. 70)

All of our introjected values, derived from our regard complex, combine to form what Carl Rogers and his colleagues termed our *conditions of worth*. Conditions of worth are the values and attitudes that have become part of the way in which we see ourselves – our self-concepts. If self-actualising thwarts the actualising tendency, this may generate tension or anxiety that, if it is admitted to conscious awareness or comes close to being admitted to conscious awareness, may result in the individual seeking counselling.

Rogers credited Stanley Standal with developing the idea of *conditions of worth*. Just as Standal coined the term *unconditional positive regard* as an alternative to acceptance, so he replaced 'introjected values' with conditions of worth:

> The self-structure is characterized by a condition of worth when a self-experience or set of related self-experiences is either avoided or sought solely because the individual discriminates it as being less or more worthy of self-regard . . . A condition of worth arises when the positive regard of a significant other is conditional, when the individual feels that in some respects he is prized and in others not. Gradually this same attitude is assimilated into his own self-regard complex, and he values an experience positively or negatively solely because of these conditions of worth which he has taken over from others, not because the experience enhances or fails to enhance his organism.
>
> (Rogers 1959: p. 209)

If *unconditional* positive regard is experienced, then valuing may be based on an internal locus of evaluation (that is, on whether or not the experiencing maintains or enhances the organism). However, if valuing is based on values 'adopted' from others, then there is no reference to organismic valuing. This in turn links with symbolisation, for if I value an experience (as positive or negative) as if it were referenced to my own actualising tendency when in fact my referencing is 'second hand' (that is, to values introjected from others), then my symbolisation is inaccurate. In other words:

> An experience may be perceived as organismically satisfying, when in fact this is not true. Thus a condition of worth, because it disturbs the valuing process, prevents the individual from functioning freely and with maximum effectiveness.
>
> (Rogers 1959: p. 210)

When there is a discrepancy between *organismic experiencing* and the *self as perceived*, the individual is in a state of *incongruence* – that is, the physiological organism and conscious awareness are not coexisting in harmony:

> When such a discrepancy exists, the state is one of incongruence between self and experience. This state is one of tension and internal confusion, since in some respects the individual's behavior will be regulated by the actualizing tendency, and in other respects by the

self-actualizing tendency, thus producing discordant or incomprehens-
ible behaviors.

(Rogers 1959: p. 203)

Note again the crucial distinction between the actualising tendency and self-actualising.

When the individual is incongruent, the term *vulnerability* is used to describe
the potentialities of this state, and when individuals are not consciously aware of
this incongruence, they are:

> potentially vulnerable to anxiety, threat, and disorganization. If a
> significant new experience demonstrates the discrepancy so clearly
> that it must be consciously perceived, then the individual will be
> threatened, and his concept of self disorganized by this contradictory
> and unassimilable experience.
>
> (Rogers 1959: p. 204)

A consequence of experiencing anxiety because the concept of self and actual
experience are incongruent is the *defensive* psychological processes of *denial* or
distortion. *Self*-actualising demands that we maintain and enhance the way that
we see ourselves – the tendency is to both maintain and enhance the *self-concept*.
So the concept of self must be *defended* against anything that is potentially
threatening to it.

Carl Rogers defined *anxiety* as:

> a state of uneasiness or tension whose cause is unknown. From an
> external frame of reference, anxiety is a state in which the incon-
> gruence between the concept of self and the total experience of the
> individual is approaching symbolization in awareness. When experi-
> ence is *obviously* discrepant from the self-concept, a defensive response
> to threat becomes increasingly difficult. Anxiety is the response of the
> organism to the 'subception' that such discrepancy may enter aware-
> ness, thus forcing a change in the self-concept.
>
> (Rogers 1959: p. 204)

Threat, on the other hand, occurs when there is an experiencing (a perception or
anticipation) of incongruence:

> If we think of the structure of the self as being a symbolic elaboration
> of a portion of the private experiential world of the organism, we may
> realize that when much of this private world is denied symbolization,
> certain basic tensions result. We find, then, that there is a very real
> discrepancy between the experiencing organism as it exists, and the
> concept of self which exerts such a governing influence on behavior.
> This self is now very inadequately representative of the experience of
> the organism. Conscious control becomes more difficult as the organ-
> ism strives to satisfy needs which are not consciously admitted, and to
> react to experiences which are denied by the conscious self. Tension
> then exists, and if the individual becomes to any degree aware of this
> tension or discrepancy, he feels anxious, feels that he is not united or
> integrated, that he is unsure of his direction.
>
> (Rogers 1951: pp. 510–11)

Thus *self-actualising* demands that the concept of self be *defended* against any perceived threats to it:

> Defense is the behavioral response of the organism to threat, the goal of which is the maintenance of the current structure of the self. This goal is achieved by the perceptual distortion of the experience in awareness, in such a way as to reduce the incongruity between the experience and the structure of the self, or by the denial to awareness of an experience, thus denying any threat to the self. Defensiveness is the term denoting a state in which the behaviors are of the sort described.
>
> (Rogers 1959: pp. 204–5)

The two main processes of defence in client-centred personality theory are those in which experiences may be *denied* accurate symbolisation in our awareness, and those in which they may be granted only a *distorted* symbolisation. (Incidentally, another way of understanding what is meant by 'symbolisation' might be to consider the notion of *pre*-symbolisation! You know that feeling you get when there is something niggling away yet you 'can't quite put your finger on it'? Well, when it feels evasive or illusive it has yet to be accurately symbolised in awareness – and when you *have* put your finger on it, you have symbolised it in your awareness.)

If an experience is threatening to the concept of self, it may be *denied* entry to conscious awareness as a way of defending the self, and the more important our self-beliefs are to us, the more rigid and tough will be our defences against any threats to them. Another defensive option that the self has is to permit experiencing into awareness, yet only in a *distorted* fashion. In other words, the organism cannot deny crying because the tears felt real, wet and salty enough. However, they were shed because someone nearby must have been peeling onions or some grit had found its way into the eye socket, or the person has a cold coming on – they were not due to any distress:

> I gradually came to realize that one denies awareness – which seemed to me a better term than repression – to those feelings which do not fit into the current concept of self. If I see myself in such and such a fashion – as poor at mathematics, for example – and I find myself solving a mathematical problem, well, that was luck, or chance. That wasn't me. I have to deny or distort in my awareness things that don't fit my concept of self . . . The self-concept becomes a sort of screening device, determining what is admitted to awareness.
>
> (Rogers and Russell 2002: p. 248)

There is also a notion of psychological defence known as *pre-perception* or '*subception*', which is the non-conscious denial of experience to awareness. Experimental support for this notion arose from the flashing of subliminal images in front of volunteers who were wired up to various physiological measuring devices. If, for instance, an individual was scared of spiders, there was a measurable physiological reaction to the image of a spider even though the picture was flashed on screen more quickly than the eye could see. In other words, an experience that is *subceived* (or pre-perceived) as threatening to the self may be denied to awareness without the individual even being consciously aware of threats to their self-concept or their defensive psychological processes.

> We feel internally threatened when we recognize that something we're experiencing – anger or hatred or positive feelings, something that we're denying to awareness – is getting close to awareness. And there, the concept of *subception*, which was to my mind pretty well confirmed by our research, was a very valuable concept. Without any conscious awareness, one can *subceive* certain things in the environment. That's true physically; it's also true psychologically: one could subceive the fact that 'I am unhappy in my marriage' or that 'I don't like my mother', or whatever. And it's then that a person feels anxious because the experience one is having is almost breaking through into the concept of self.
>
> (Rogers and Russell 2002: p. 252)

Carl Rogers summarised much of this when he wrote:

> It may help to clarify this basic concept of incongruence if we recognize that several of the terms we are defining are simply different vantage points for viewing this phenomenon. If an individual is in a state of incongruence between self and experience and we are looking at him from an external point of view, we see him as vulnerable (if he is unaware of the discrepancy) or threatened (if he has some awareness of it). If we are viewing him from a social point of view, then this incongruence is psychological maladjustment. If the individual is viewing himself, he may even see himself as adjusted (if he has no awareness of the discrepancy) or anxious (if he dimly subceives it) or threatened or disorganized (if the discrepancy has forced itself upon his awareness).
>
> (Rogers 1959: p. 204)

Another fundamental aspect of client-centred personality theory is that *experiencing remains available to conscious awareness given the right conditions*, and especially given the relative absence of threat to the self-concept (there therefore being less need to defend the self). When writing of this, Carl Rogers mentioned that he was aware of the pressure of the seat on his buttocks. Say this in a group and suddenly *everyone* will become aware of the pressure on their own buttocks (and indeed you may well have become aware of the pressure on your own buttocks as you read this last sentence). Thus the organismic experience of sitting is *being experienced* and although not necessarily in awareness, it is nevertheless *available to awareness*.

There are those who argue that because Carl was so passionate about client-centred therapy (and the person-centred approach) as *a way of being*, learning and understanding theory is therefore not really necessary at all – that if the individual can *be* (or strive with some success to be) the therapist (or core) conditions, client-centred *theory* is almost an irrelevance. Such arguments are sometimes supported by comments written by Rogers early in his career, such as the following:

> I might at [this] point say a word or two about theory. I remember very clearly telling my students at Ohio State, 'I have no use for psycho-

logical theory'. Later I came to change that point of view, but I realized eventually that I had no use for psychological theory which was not my own . . . So I really thought that I had no use for psychological theory. Later I came to realize its significance.

(Rogers and Russell 2002: pp. 246–7)

Please note the phrase 'Later I came to change that point of view . . . Later I came to realize its significance'! These very same people who dismiss theory often also claim that they engage as *whole* persons with other *whole* persons, yet somehow see no contradiction whatsoever when omitting a significant part (that is, *theory*) from the *whole* that is client-centred therapy. Yet how do we *understand* or *empathise* with another person? It is very clear indeed that to Rogers both unconditional positive regard and empathic understanding need to be integrated and deeply held beliefs and values residing within the client-centred therapist, and that congruence means the absence of denial or distortion with regard to any significant aspects of self-experience. To perceive another person means to filter the 'stimuli' from them through our own feelings and meanings – and if a client-centred way of being is deeply integrated, those sensations and meanings will include cognitive as well as emotional and physiological dimensions. So many students of Rogers have made comments along the lines of 'I was searching for something, and when I picked up and read a book by Carl Rogers, it *spoke* to me. Here, at last, was someone who seemed to understand what it *feels* like to be me, what it *means* to be me'. Perhaps this kind of comment is only to be expected. After all, *we taught Carl Rogers all that he knew.* Client-centred theory grew out of listening to and striving to understand hundreds upon hundreds of clients, and in turn that theory can now inform how we continue to strive to understand one another.

Lest there be any misunderstanding, it is not the contention here that client-centred therapists are fully aware of theory when meeting with clients. The client-centred therapist experiencing 'Aha! – that sounded like an introjected value' or 'Hmm, this subceived threat to the concept of self is clearly distorted in symbolisation' would hardly be paying extraordinary attention to the client's world of feelings and personal meanings! Rather:

There needs to be an intellectual context into which what he or she is doing fits.

(Rogers and Russell 2002: p. 272)

This is not to say, though, that such issues as introjection, subception, threat, self-concept, distortion, symbolisation and so on are altogether irrelevant, for it might be useful and appropriate to make links with theory in supervision or in discussion with colleagues. However, our knowledge (hopefully or ideally derived from experiential, person-centred learning) is unarguably a significant part of our whole being, guiding and informing us even if in non-conscious ways, or in ways that are less prominent than or secondary to our integrated embodiment of the therapist conditions.

In illustration of the relevance of client-centred *theory* to client-centred *practice*, person-centred *supervision* has as a primary focus the extent to which the therapist is able to *be* the core conditions in the counselling relationship. It might, for example, be helpful for the therapist to reflect upon the nature of a particular client's defensive processes, to explore whether significant client experiencing might be denied to or distorted in awareness. After all, clients are unlikely even to seek therapy unless they are incongruent. Thus person-centred supervision is an opportunity to give more prominence to client-centred theory than would be the case in therapy itself, and through doing so the therapist might just become more open to experiencing that client more fully. The therapist is usually (and ideally) so closely attuned to *client* experiencing *in the moment*, and *moment by moment*, that self-reflecting activities and supervision are a wonderful opportunity to explore more deeply the therapist's own experiencing and underpinning values, attitudes, beliefs and practices, with a view to maintaining and enhancing the quality of presence of the therapist conditions. An understanding of incongruence is invaluable and indispensable in terms of maximising therapist congruence, more deeply experiencing unconditional positive regard, and empathically understanding the nature of the whole person that is the client – and the therapist.

Empathy and therapist congruence

> The order in which these therapeutic conditions are described has some significance because they are logically intertwined. In the first place, the therapist must achieve a strong, accurate empathy. But such deep sensitivity to the moment-to-moment 'being' of another person requires that the therapist first accept, and to some degree prize, the other person. That is to say, a sufficiently strong empathy can hardly exist without a considerable degree of unconditional positive regard. However, since neither of these conditions can possibly be meaningful in the relationship unless they are real, the therapist must be, both in these respects and in others, integrated and genuine within the therapeutic encounter. Therefore, it seems to me that genuineness or congruence is the most basic of the three conditions.
>
> (Rogers 1989: p. 11)

The third, fourth and fifth necessary and sufficient conditions (congruence, unconditional positive regard and empathic understanding) became known as the *core conditions* of client-centred therapy; others have called these the *therapist conditions*. At various times in his career Carl Rogers was asked which of these core conditions was the most important. Here is one version he gave about *congruence* in 1975:

> In the ordinary interactions of life – between marital and sex partners, between teacher and student, employer and employee, or between colleagues, it is probable that congruence is the most important element. Such genuineness involves letting the other person know 'where you are' emotionally. It may involve confrontation, and the personally owned and straightforward expression of both negative and positive feelings. Thus congruence is a basis for living together in a climate of realness.
>
> (Rogers 1975: p. 9)

One definition of congruence is that the two shapes of the *whole organism* and that differentiated part of it which is known as the *self* correspond (the actualising tendency and self-actualising being as one) – that is, when our experiencing and our perceptions of that experiencing are in harmony. Congruence, then, is described as a *state* – the 'state' is that either the two shapes do overlap exactly, or they do not.

Some writers have defined this 'accurate overlap' of organism and self, or experience and the perceiving of that experience, as meaning that the congruent therapist's 'outward' communications are consistent with their inner sensations and meanings. Although this makes sense and is to some extent true, it is also only part of the whole picture. For instance, if therapist A's inner feeling is a fatigued disinterest linked with personal meanings (including values) about boredom, and the outward expression of this is to say 'I am bored', then therapist A could be deemed to be being congruent. However, it would also be true to say that the congruence of therapist A does not evidence a great deal of unconditional positive regard or empathic understanding as deeply embedded and integrated personal characteristics. For therapist A to voice boredom without having accessed (that is, in *denial* of) client-centred attitudes, beliefs and values could be deemed to be more representative of a state of *incongruence*. Now therapist B steps in and does not communicate any feeling of boredom because to do so would hardly be client-centred. Is therapist B congruent? Not necessarily! If the feelings and meanings of fatigued disinterest through boredom are denied access to awareness (and hence cannot be voiced) because they would be too threatening to therapist B's self-concept (therapist B's self-concept is of being a *good* client-centred practitioner), then therapist B is also incongruent. Therapist C has an awareness of feeling tired and losing interest, yet also accesses a deeply held client-centred way of being, and will make a choice about whether or not to voice boredom depending upon the outcome of processing *both* significant experiences and their meanings. Again, there are those who seem to see congruence as meaning 'harmony' because the two shapes of organism and self correspond. In fact, *being congruent might mean embracing conflict* – conflict that is usually avoided through psychological processes of denial and distortion. Gradational rather than 'black-and-white' thinking (pertinent to *extensionality*, which as we shall see shortly was considered by Rogers to be one of the five ingredients of congruence) might mean *being many things simultaneously*:

> It is not simple to achieve such reality. Being real involves the difficult task of being acquainted with the flow of experiencing going on within oneself, a flow marked especially by complexity and continuous change.
>
> (Rogers 1989: pp. 11–13)

Returning to the theme of the therapist voicing to a client a feeling of boredom in that client's presence, Carl stated that during such moments he would strive to remain in ongoing touch with his own *changing* feelings and meanings. For instance, he would *own* his feeling of boredom ('own' in the sense that he would view his feeling as his own feeling, and not as some putative 'fact' about the client). Nor is this feeling of boredom fixed, rigid or permanent, nor does it exist in isolation. (This might be an example of what is meant by *extensionality* as a feature of congruence – boredom is an abstraction from the whole. This is not a boring client and nor is the boredom continuous.) Rogers would include in his verbalisation his discomfort in expressing his feeling of boredom and his distress at even feeling it and, as he does so, he realises that actually 'behind' this *apparent* boredom is a feeling of distance between himself and the client, and that he would wish for greater proximity. This, too, is voiced, and he would most definitely not feel bored as he eagerly (and with some apprehension) awaited the client's reactions to such disclosures:

> I also feel a new sensitivity to him now that I have shared this feeling which has been a barrier between us. I am far more able to hear the surprise, or perhaps the hurt, in his voice as he now finds himself speaking more genuinely because I have dared to be real with him. I have let myself be a person – real, imperfect – in my relationship with him.
>
> (Rogers 1989: p. 12)

While ideally it might be considered best if the therapist experienced no (apparently) negative feelings at all towards clients (although Rogers was honest enough to say that he thought all therapists did experience negative feelings or thoughts about their clients from time to time), Carl Rogers believed that when they are present it can be more harmful to keep them hidden than to voice them. Although such negative feelings might at first glance seem potentially harmful or damaging to clients, congruence is a better policy than dishonesty, pretence and false posturing.

> It is not easy for a client, or for any human being, to entrust his most deeply shrouded feelings to another person. It is even more difficult for a disturbed person to share his deepest and most troubling feelings with a therapist. The genuineness of the therapist is one of the elements in the relationship that make the risk of sharing easier and less fraught with dangers.
>
> (Rogers 1989: p. 13)

We shall see when we explore therapeutic process in Chapter 5 that one phase is the discovery that the core of the personality is positive – likeable. If we can trust that at heart clients are inherently positive, perhaps congruent therapists can have a similar faith in themselves. If I know myself and am aware of what lies within me, I can come to know that fuelling my apparently negative or hostile feelings are more understandable and acceptable features of my being. Thus the more I have engaged in my own self-development activities, the less likely it is that I will have to discover my potential through and with clients.

Being many things simultaneously might be illustrated by looking at the notions of *self-as-object* and *self-as-process*. George Kelly (Kelly 1955) wrote about *personal constructs*, and more recently Dave Mearns (Mearns 2002) has written about *configurations of self* – a phrase coined by Carl Rogers in his 1959 paper. Just as Rogers differentiated between *self-concept* (how individuals see themselves) and *self-structure* (how individuals see themselves viewed by another person), so *individuals* can view aspects of *themselves*. Suppose that person A is a mother of two children who is training to become a client-centred therapist. One 'personal construct' that she may have is composed around parenting. Another configuration of self is constructed around being a student. Person A can look at each of these constructs, and in doing so they become somewhat objectified – hence *self-as-object*. Indeed, she could draw diagrams of each of these constructs, mapping and charting their relevant components. Now suppose that on a training day one of her children feels a little ill – not dramatically ill, just slightly poorly. The 'good mother' personal construct tells her to miss out on a day's training in order to care for her child, yet her 'good student' configuration tells her to attend her course. Thus there is a conflict *between two of the self-structures* of person A. Every individual is made up of far more than just two personal constructs or configurations – and let us not forget organismic valuing either! However, there is also the *self-as-process* to consider. If it is possible to identify and examine aspects of the self-structure, what about *the self that is doing the exploring*? In the previous example of therapists A, B and C, only therapist C really utilised self-as-process. Therapist A was influenced only by a tired, bored aspect of self, and therapist B was influenced only by client-centred conditions of worth. It is the *self-as-process* that enables access to *all* significant configurations of self *and* organismic valuing, and the self-as-process that is free to make informed choices based on the sensory and visceral evidence available to it.

> I have learned that my total organismic sensing of a situation is more trustworthy than my intellect . . . I have found that when I have trusted some inner non-intellectual sensing, I have discovered wisdom in the move . . . As I gradually come to trust my total reactions more deeply, I find that I can use them to guide my thinking . . . I think of it as trusting the totality of my experience, which I have learned to suspect is wiser than my intellect. It is fallible I am sure, but I believe it to be less fallible than my conscious mind alone.
>
> (Rogers 1961: pp. 22–3)

Two other common misunderstandings occur, both concerning the 'communication' of congruence. All too often it seems to be 'forgotten' that therapist communication of congruence (or client perception of therapist congruence, even to a minimal degree) was *not* one of the original (1957 or 1959) necessary and sufficient conditions. It is necessary (and sufficient) only that the client perceives the unconditional positive regard and empathic understanding of the therapist as being genuine. The crucial importance of congruence is that the unconditional positive regard and empathic understanding of the therapist are real – that is, authentic and genuine. There can be nothing more inaccurate or misleading than the notion of 'communicating congruence' for, as we have seen, congruence means a state of being wherein there is no denial to awareness or distorted symbolisation in awareness of significant sensory or visceral experiencing. Imagine therapist D 'communicating congruence' (and think about how therapeutic it might be for the client) by saying to that client 'Right now I am neither denying symbolisation of significant sensory or visceral experience to my awareness, nor granting only a distorted symbolisation in my awareness of significant sensory or visceral experiencing'! Personally, I would rather see a different counsellor! Maybe therapist C.

Yet none of this is intended to detract from the following:

> Being genuine also involves the willingness to be and to express, in my words and my behavior, the various feelings and attitudes which exist

in me. It is only in this way that the relationship can have *reality*, and reality seems deeply important as a first condition. It is only by providing the genuine reality which is in me, that the other person can successfully seek for the reality in him. I have found this to be true even when the attitudes I feel are not attitudes with which I am pleased, or attitudes which seem conducive to a good relationship. It seems extremely important to be *real*.

(Rogers 1961: p. 33)

It may be worth remembering that a congruent communication of an attitude with which the therapist does not feel pleased could well include the feeling of displeasure that accompanies the attitude.

Carl Rogers defined congruence as a *cluster of factors* that included *congruence of self and experience, openness to experience, psychological adjustment, extensionality* and *maturity*.

The first aspect of congruence is *congruence of self and experience*, typified by individuals who constantly revise and reorganise their concept of self to include characteristics that would previously have been inconsistent with self:

Thus when self-experiences are accurately symbolized, and are included in the self-concept in this accurately symbolized form, then the state is one of congruence of self and experience. If this were completely true of all self-experiences, the individual would be a fully functioning person . . . If it is true of some specific aspect of experience, such as the individual's experience in a given relationship or in a given moment of time, then we can say that the individual is to this degree in a state of congruence. Other terms which are in a general way synonymous are these: integrated, whole, genuine.

(Rogers 1959: p. 206)

Openness to experience, the second factor, occurs when the self-structure experiences no threat to itself. In other words, openness to experience is the exact opposite of defensiveness:

whether the stimulus is the impact of a configuration of form, color, or sound in the environment on the sensory nerves, or a memory trace from the past, or a visceral sensation of fear, pleasure, or disgust, it is completely available to the individual's awareness. In the hypothetical person who is completely open to his experience, his concept of self would be a symbolization in awareness which would be completely congruent with his experience. There would, therefore, be no possibility of threat.

(Rogers 1959: p. 206)

In other words, complete and total openness to experience would only be possible if there was also a complete absence of denial and distortion.

Thirdly, *psychological adjustment* means that:

the concept of the self is such that all experiences are or may be assimilated on a symbolic level into the gestalt of the self-structure. Optimal psychological adjustment is thus synonymous with complete congruence of self and experience, or complete openness to experience. On the practical level, improvement in psychological adjustment is equivalent to progress toward this end point.

(Rogers 1959: p. 206)

If there is a complete absence of denial and distortion, the individual experiences no threat and there is therefore no need to feel either vulnerable or anxious.

Extensionality is the fourth ingredient of congruence, and it is a term derived from general semantics, meaning that the individual is aware that any experience is an *abstraction* from the whole and not the whole itself (the map is not the territory, for instance), and thus abstractions are by their very nature limited and differentiated (a fairly comprehensive and novel view of general semantics can be found in the 'Null-A' science fiction books written by AE van Vogt). The extensional individual will give 'pride of place' to facts rather than concepts, and will be aware that such facts are 'anchored' in space and time (as in 'what is true today might not be so true tomorrow'), evaluation is multiple and varied (gradational, not simply 'left or right' or 'black or white' or 'right or wrong'), and inferences and abstractions will be constantly tested against reality.

The fifth and final component in this congruence cluster is *maturity*, defined by Carl Rogers as meaning that the person:

> perceives realistically and in an extensional manner, is not defensive, accepts the responsibility of being different from others, accepts responsibility for his own behavior, evaluates experience in terms of the evidence coming from his own senses, changes his evaluation of experience only on the basis of new evidence, accepts others as unique individuals different from himself, prizes himself, and prizes others. If his behavior has these characteristics, then there will automatically follow all the types of behavior which are more popularly thought of as constituting psychological maturity.

(Rogers 1959: p. 207)

In summary, Rogers wrote:

> Congruence is the term which defines the state. Openness to experience is the way an internally congruent individual meets new experience. Psychological adjustment is congruence as viewed from a social point of view. Extensional is the term which describes the specific types of behavior of a congruent individual. Maturity is a broader term describing the personality characteristics and behavior of a person who is, in general, congruent.

(Rogers 1959: p. 207)

So congruence is a state of being comprised of several factors. If the *direct communication of congruence* is utterly irrelevant, might there nevertheless be issues about *congruent communications*? The answer is yes, because in terms of the 'core' conditions for client-centred therapy, congruence was originally placed first of the three *because of the critical importance of both unconditional positive regard and empathic understanding being authentic* and being *perceived by the client as genuine*. We have seen that when writing of psychological adjustment, Carl Rogers stated that 'On the practical level, improvement in psychological adjustment is equivalent to progress toward this end point'. The would-be client-centred therapist, then, is likely to engage in processes that aim to optimise the likelihood of therapist congruence in counselling relationships.

The therapist who passes judgements, evaluates, diagnoses, praises, gives opinions, reassures and problem solves (and so on) may well be being congruent. However, unconditional positive regard (in particular) and empathic under-standing do not feature as prominent or primary components of this particular congruence. Therapists who, for instance, tell their clients what they would do if faced with a similar situation may well be being 'real' and genuine. However, 'transparency' in client-centred therapy means that the client will see uncondi-tional positive regard and empathic understanding residing at the heart of the therapist's presence. In client-centred therapy there is no professional counselling façade or mask. The 'naked' or 'uncovered truth' reveals unconditional positive regard and empathy as deeply embedded and integrated aspects of the therapist's way of being.

Within this client-centred way of being, congruence is described as a *state* (whereas unconditional positive regard is seen as an *attitude*, and empathic understanding as a *process*). Congruence can be viewed as a *state of being* because at any given moment the person either is or is not congruent, or more accurately, could be located somewhere along the continuum between absolute congruence and total incongruence. However, this does not have to mean that congruence is a *fixed* or *static* state. Indeed Carl Rogers said that if this were so there would be no client-centred therapists at all!

> Another point worth noting is that the stress is upon the experience *in the relationship*. It is not to be expected that the therapist is a completely congruent person at all times. Indeed if this were a necessary condition there would be no therapy. But it is enough if in this particular moment of this immediate relationship with this specific person he is completely and fully himself, with his experience of the moment being accurately symbolized and integrated into the picture he holds of himself. Thus it is that imperfect human beings can be of therapeutic assistance to other imperfect human beings.
>
> (Rogers 1959: p. 215)

It is a condition, then, that *during the therapy session* client-centred counsellors strive to be as congruent as it is possible for them to be, to come as close to the ideal of congruence as is possible. Concluding that in terms of any given moment congruence is a *state*, and that client-centred therapists strive to maximise and *be* in that state during counselling sessions, does not have to mean that there are no *process* dimensions to congruence. We might ask, for example, what factors and activities might be conducive to maximising congruence during the therapy session. Perhaps a few possibilities might be worth mentioning here.

If therapist A in the recent example could be seen as congruent but not especially client-centred, and if therapist A would like to work towards becoming more client-centred, then looking for ways of developing authentic (that is, congruent) attitudes and beliefs that value the dignity, capacity and potential resources of the client (as explored further when looking at unconditional positive regard) might make sense. Carl Rogers wrote that we need to *permit* ourselves to be empathic with another, adding that the word 'permit' may seem strange to many, for:

> Our first reaction to most of the statements which we hear from other people is an immediate evaluation, cause or judgment, rather than an understanding of it. When someone expresses some feeling or attitude or belief, our tendency is, almost immediately, to feel 'That's right', or 'That's stupid', 'That's abnormal', 'That's unreasonable', 'That's incorrect', 'That's not nice'. Very rarely do we permit ourselves to *understand* precisely what the meaning of his statement is to him. I believe this is because understanding is risky. If I let myself really understand another person, I might be changed by that understanding. And we all fear change. So as I say, it is not an easy thing to permit oneself to understand an individual, to enter thoroughly and completely and empathically into his frame of reference. It is also a rare thing.
>
> (Rogers 1961: p. 18)

Thus a link between congruence and empathic understanding is *danger*, for personal (that is, *therapist*) change will in all likelihood be a consequence of accurate empathic understanding of clients. Unless therapists are open to the possibility of personal change *to themselves* through engaging in counselling *as the counsellor*, empathic understanding would be threatening to the concept of self (and hence the self would strive to defend itself against this threat). Thus we can see the vital importance of *therapist self-development*, for Rogers wrote of being empathic:

> In some sense it means that you lay aside your self; this can only be done by persons who are secure enough in themselves that they know they will not get lost in what may turn out to be the strange or bizarre world of the other, and that they can comfortably return to their own world when they wish.
>
> (Rogers 1980: p. 143)

Rogers saying that *in some sense* therapists 'set aside their self' may well be significant. Perhaps it is symptomatic of the shift from a 'total' laying aside of the self (1951), to greater therapist transparency (during the 'intervening years'), to eventual modification into the self being disciplined around respect and empathy (1987).

In other words, the congruence of a client-centred therapist includes both an openness to the possibility of being changed oneself through offering therapy *and* the personal strength and inner security to boldly (yet sensitively) go where no one has gone before – often not even the client – safe in the knowledge that there is a way back.

> I know that I have some knowledge of who I am, so I can let myself go into the world of this other person – even though it's a frightening, crazy, bizarre world – because I know I can come back to my world and be myself. When one is not very secure in oneself, one can get tangled into the world of the other and not know who's who. That's a very painful situation.
>
> (Rogers and Russell 2002: p. 281)

There are many ways in which Carl Rogers linked therapist congruence and empathic understanding with a journey of personal growth for the therapist. For instance, empathic understanding is a quality that the therapist *offers*, rather than something that is drawn from the therapist by specific types of clients or concerns. If empathy comes more easily with certain clients or problems, the therapist is *evaluating* and *judgemental* (and certainly not unconditional), so *becoming non-evaluative* is a major aspect of the journey towards becoming a congruent client-centred therapist. How might someone learn to become less judgemental? It is perhaps the case that each and every (trainee) client-centred therapist needs to find ways of achieving both broad (social, political and cultural, for instance) and personal (through receiving therapy or engaging in equivalent activities them-selves and through counselling practice) understanding of human nature – and although Carl Rogers shunned the mantle of 'guru', there is nevertheless much to learn from studying his work.

It is also helpful if the therapist is authentically interested in the other person, demonstrating 'an extraordinary kind of concentrated attention' (Rogers 1951: p. 349). So often in training groups, for instance, student A speaks and student B says something about their own experience or thoughts, with the consequence that student A feels completely unheard, and wonders whether it was worth saying anything at all in the first place. Students C and D then pitch in with *their* own thoughts, feelings and experiences, so actually *no one* feels heard or that there is even an attempt to value the speakers by striving to understand them. As Rogers said, 'Without attention there can be no understanding and hence no communication' (Rogers 1951: p. 349) – and this means *paying attention to the client's world of feelings and meanings*. Yes, congruence *does* include therapists being aware of their inner flow of sensations and meanings. However, if the therapist's attention is either focused on one specific point that has significance *to the therapist* or is devoted to how the therapist will *respond*, then he or she is not attending as fully as possible to the client, and 'this is not communication in any sense of the word' (Rogers 1951: p. 349). Linked with therapist unconditional positive regard, the client-centred therapist conveys an *authentic* valuing of clients in part through this precious attention to the *client's* world of feelings and personal meanings.

> The accuracy of the therapist's empathic understanding has often been emphasised, but more important is the therapist's *interest* in appreciat-ing the world of the client and offering such understanding with the willingness to be corrected. This creates a process in which the therapist gets closer and closer to the client's meanings and feelings, developing an ever-deepening relationship based on respect for and understanding of the other person.
>
> (Rogers and Raskin 1989: p. 171)

Thus the journey towards becoming a client-centred therapist involves the development of a *genuine desire* to respect others through paying attention to them – not 'laying aside your own self' because *Carl Rogers* or a *facilitator* says that this is how it should be. A genuine desire will be integrated and fully present and will be based upon the internal locus of evaluation of the therapist rather than being a value that is introjected from some significant other – not even Rogers. Another way of putting this is that *therapist* needs for positive regard and positive self-regard based on introjected values are not the sole determinants of *client-centred* therapist behaviour.

However, respect goes two ways, for Carl Rogers believed that *therapist self-respect* was an important factor, too. Having stated the importance of being able to enter the private world of another without becoming 'lost' in it, he furthered this thinking when he wrote:

> Can I be strong enough as a person to be separate from the other? Can I be a sturdy respecter of my own feelings, my own needs, as well as his? Can I own and, if need be, express my own feelings as something belonging to me and separate from his feelings? Am I strong enough in my own separateness that I will not be downcast by his depression, frightened by his fear, nor engulfed by his dependency? Is my inner self hardy enough to realise that I am not destroyed by his anger, taken over by his need for dependence, nor enslaved by his love, but that I exist separate from him with feelings and rights of my own? When I can freely feel this strength of being a separate person, then I find that I can let myself go much more deeply in understanding and accepting him because I am not fearful of losing myself.
>
> (Rogers 1961: p. 52)

Client-centred therapist congruence therefore includes personal strength and robust self-respect – a capacity to absorb the strong feelings of another without either being threatened by or drowning in them, or being 'seduced' into meeting the needs of the other. Carl continued:

> The next question is closely related. Am I secure enough within myself to permit him his separateness? Can I permit him to be what he is – honest or deceitful, infantile or adult, despairing or over-confident? Can I give him the freedom to be? Or do I feel that he should follow my advice, or remain somewhat dependent on me, or mould himself after me? In this connection think of the interesting small study by Parson which found that the less well-adjusted and less competent counsellor tends to induce conformity to himself, to have clients who model themselves after him. On the other hand, the better-adjusted and more competent counsellor can interact with a client through many interviews without interfering with the freedom of the client to develop a personality quite separate from that of his therapist. I should prefer to be in this latter class, whether as parent or supervisor or counsellor.
>
> (Rogers 1961: pp. 52–3)

If an element of a therapist's self-concept is 'knowing the way' for clients, then that therapist is likely to lead clients, advise them, foster dependency or even see him- or herself as a role model to be copied, followed and admired. Therefore a crucial factor in client-centred therapist congruence is not only the strength and self-respect that enables 'uncluttered' entry to the world of the other, but also the strength to permit the other person the dignity of being whoever it is that they are.

To the therapist, it is a new venture in relating. He feels, 'Here is this other person, my client. I'm a little afraid of him, afraid of the depths in him as I am a little afraid of the depths in myself. Yet as he speaks, I begin to feel a respect for him, to feel my kinship to him. I sense how frightening his world is for him, how tightly he tries to hold it in place. I would like to sense his feelings, and I would like him to know that I understand his feelings. I would like him to know that I stand with him in his tight, constricted little world, and that I can look upon it relatively unafraid. Perhaps I can make it a safer world for him. I would like my feelings in this relationship with him to be as clear and transparent as possible, so that they are a discernible reality for him, to which he can return again and again. I would like to go with him on the fearful journey into himself, into the buried fear, and hate, and love which he has never been able to let flow in him. I recognise that this is a very human and unpredictable journey for me, as well as for him, and that I may, without even knowing my fear, shrink away within myself from some of the feelings he discovers. To this extent I know I will be limited in my ability to help him. I realise that at times his own fears may make him perceive me as uncaring, as rejecting, as an intruder, as one who does not understand. I want fully to accept these feelings in him, and yet I hope also that my own real feelings will show through so clearly that in time he cannot fail to perceive them. Most of all I want him to encounter in me a real person. I do not need to be uneasy as to whether my own feelings are 'therapeutic'. What I am and what I feel are good enough to be a basis for therapy, if I can transparently *be* what I am and what I feel in relationship to him. Then perhaps he can be what he is, openly and without fear.'

(Rogers 1961: pp. 66–7)

As well as self-respect as a constituent of therapist congruence, *self-understanding* is absolutely crucial, too. To be authentic means that:

no inner barriers keep him from sensing what it feels like to be the client at each moment of the relationship; and that he can convey something of his empathic understanding to the client. It means that the therapist has been comfortable in entering this relationship fully, without knowing cognitively where it will lead, satisfied with providing a climate which will permit the client the utmost freedom to become himself.

(Rogers 1961: p. 185)

Carl Rogers wrote of intercultural work, stating how 'I understand your feelings but I've never personally oppressed you' or 'I can understand because I've been oppressed, too' may be natural responses to disadvantaged people, but such expressions are of no help whatsoever. Effectiveness for Rogers needed to include:

the realisation and ownership of 'I think white'. For men trying to deal with women's rage, it may be helpful for the man to recognise 'I think male'. In spite of all our efforts to seem unprejudiced, we actually carry within us many prejudiced attitudes.

Rage needs to be *heard*. This does not mean that it simply needs to be listened to. It needs to be accepted, taken within, and understood empathically. While the diatribes and accusations appear to be deliberate attempts to hurt the whites – an act of catharsis to dissolve centuries of abuse, oppression, and injustice – the truth about rage is that it only dissolves when it is really heard and understood, without reservations. Afterwards, the blacks or other minority members change in what seems a miraculous way, as though a weight has been lifted from their shoulders.

To achieve this kind of empathic listening the white needs to listen to his own feelings, too, his feelings of anger and resentment at 'unjust' accusations. At some point he too will need to express these, but the primary task is to enter empathically the minority world of hate and bitterness and resentment and to know that world as an understandable, acceptable part of reality.

(Rogers 1978: pp. 133–4)

There is also a *'practice makes perfect'* element to therapist personal growth, as Rogers believed that:

Experienced therapists offer a higher degree of empathy to their clients than those less experienced . . . Evidently, therapists do learn, as the years go by, to come closer to their ideal of a therapist and to be more sensitively understanding.

(Rogers 1980, p. 148)

Stating that this journey of personal growth 'puts a heavy demand on the therapist as a person', Rogers, albeit with some discomfort, reluctantly concluded (as had Bergin and Jasper, and Bergin and Solomon) that those therapists who felt relaxed and confident in interpersonal relationships offer greater empathic understanding than therapists who are less well integrated. Rogers wrote of counsellor training (Bergin and Jasper 1969; Bergin and Solomon 1970):

If the student is to become a therapist, the more he has been able to achieve of empathic experiencing with other individuals, the better will his preparations be. There are undoubtedly countless avenues to this end.

(Rogers 1951: p. 437)

Thus the process of becoming more congruent can be a broad-ranging activity, including the study of anthropology, sociology, cultural studies, gender studies, politics, literature, role taking in dramatic productions ('method acting'), and humanistic psychology courses. However, Carl Rogers also wrote that only rarely does *reading* something change behaviour to a significant degree, and that study was therefore not the only way of learning to become more integrated:

It can come simply through the process of living, when a sensitive person desires to understand the viewpoint and attitudes of another.

(Rogers 1951: p. 437)

'Have an open mind', 'try out something client-centred (or person-centred) experientially, if only in a small way, or even to try and prove it wrong – and judge the consequences for yourself . . .'.

But if you try them at all, you open yourself to visceral learnings that may change your behavior and change you.

(Rogers 1978: p. 103)

There has in some instances been a regrettable tendency only to define congruent as meaning transparent, real, genuine, authentic, and being without front, professional mask or façade, without mentioning the absolute necessity (and sufficiency) of the primary place of unconditional positive regard and empathic understanding within client-centred therapist congruence. Yet just about *any* practice could be justified in the name of congruence if the fundamental necessity of the other two core conditions is omitted: 'I was just being congruent . . .'.

Empathy and therapist unconditional positive regard

In the last section, we saw that Carl Rogers believed congruence to be the most important element of the 'core' conditions 'in the ordinary interactions of life'. At the same time, he said of unconditional positive regard:

But in certain other special situations, caring or prizing may turn out to be the most significant. Such situations include non-verbal relationships – parent and infant, therapist and mute psychotic, physician and very ill patient. Caring is an attitude which is known to foster creativity – a nurturing climate in which delicate, tentative new thoughts and productive processes can emerge.

(Rogers 1975: p. 9)

Unconditional positive regard is placed second in the sequence of the three therapist conditions because a 'prerequisite' is that the respect of the counsellor for a client is authentic (that is, congruent), and one of the most effective ways of communicating (or indeed of the client perceiving) unconditional positive regard is through the process of the therapist striving to empathise with and understand the client from within that client's internal frame of reference.

Carl Rogers did not commence his career in psychology with a particularly strong belief in the capacity of clients:

The more I have worked with people, both in individual therapy and in encounter groups, the more respect I've come to have for man as a person worthy of respect and a person of dignity. This value that I've come to place on the human being is something that really grows out of my experience. I didn't start with that high a regard for the individual person.

(Rogers and Evans 1975: p. 74)

In terms of *becoming* client-centred, there would appear to be a *process* along the lines of the more client-centred attitudes and beliefs are put into practice, the more meaning and strength those beliefs come to have. What might begin as a '*leap of faith*' moves toward being a more solid *belief*, which moves toward *trusting* in that belief, which moves toward a *knowing* – and client-centred therapists implement their faith–belief–trust–knowing not by *doing*, but through a way of *being*. It may well also be that the client needs to feel fully received in each phase of development in order to move on to the next one. As they enter counselling courses, trainees tend to be rather passive. As experience is gained they gradually become more inclined to listen to their clients and display some willingness to allow their clients autonomy (self-direction). However, in the early stages this passivity may be characterised by the trainee counsellor attempting to 'keep out of the way' of clients by trying to avoid any of their own feelings or thoughts straying into the session. Sometimes clients perceive this passivity as indifference rather than prizing – they might even feel rejected as they perceive their counsellor as not caring much about them, hardly seeing themselves as individuals worthy of their therapist's respect. Sadly, some counsellor training seems to be built around passivity and counsellors 'keeping out of the way', and Rogers wrote:

> This misconception of the approach has led to considerable failure in counseling – and for good reasons . . . Hence the counselor who plays a merely passive role, a listening role, may be of assistance to some clients . . . but by and large his results will be minimal, and many clients will leave, both disappointed in their failure to receive help and disgusted with the counselor for having nothing to offer.
>
> (Rogers 1951: p. 27)

We have learned that clients entering therapy are likely to be psychologically defensive because they are vulnerable and anxious. They are vulnerable and anxious because their ability to deny or distort experiencing that is threatening to their self-concept is no longer entirely successful, so there is a perceived or subceived state of tension – the client is *incongruent*. Denied or distorted experience is most likely to be permitted access to conscious awareness (and therefore be open to expression, exploration and ownership) if there is an absence or relative absence of perceived threat. Yet empathic understanding by a therapist might in itself (that is, *without* authenticity and respect) feel *very* threatening to clients. If the therapist might be thought of as an 'alter ego mirror' for a moment, then no matter how 'magical' the mirror, the client might not *want* to see or meet with their 'reflection' or 'doppelganger' (as stated in Chapter 2, in some sense there is nothing more 'confrontational' than accurate empathic understanding). If, for instance, a therapist senses that underlying a client's anger is deep pain, the client might at that moment be willing to engage with their rage yet feel really fearful of connecting with their hurt. Although it may be true that profound, sensitive and delicate empathic understanding would in this instance *include* a sensing of the client's fear of the pain that lies behind their anger, there is another crucial factor, too, namely that the therapist *respects* the client's defensive needs (prizing not prising again).

When Rogers defined congruence as a *state*, he defined unconditional positive regard as an *attitude*. This respectful attitude means a variety of things at a variety of levels. The importance of congruence is that unconditional positive regard is genuine. The importance of empathic understanding is that it is the best way to communicate unconditional positive regard and be respectful. What different meanings, then, can be ascribed to this precious and rare (because most relation-ships are conditional) attitude of *unconditional* positive regard?

First, the client-centred therapist holds a deep belief in the *actualising tendency* as the motivating force in human beings. Furthermore, the actualising tendency is viewed as trustworthy and positive, for given the right conditions people are *by nature* co-operative, social, constructive, trustworthy, creative, responsible, com-plex and fluid forward-moving entities. This fundamental acceptance of the actualising tendency as the primary human growth factor enables the client-centred therapist to see the *positive potential* in anyone and everyone. For sure, not everyone does meet with the 'right' conditions (that is, the conditions most conducive for growth), yet everyone has within them the *potential* to become all that they could be – and given the right conditions that 'becoming' will be in a positive direction.

Carl Rogers stated that his belief in the positive nature at the heart of all human beings was the single most *revolutionary* and *radical* aspect of client-centred therapy. For so long, *feelings* and *thoughts* (or at least, feelings and thoughts deemed to be antisocial, harmful, negative or just plain wrong) were considered as things to be managed, controlled, suppressed, changed, repressed, altered or influenced. From most religions through to Freudian psychoanalysis, human beings were viewed with notions of 'original sin', and unless the 'raging id' was to be controlled, the consequence would be brutal mayhem. Likewise *behaviour* was also something to be evaluated (by those who knew best, of course) and either encouraged (or reinforced), controlled (or managed) or eliminated altogether, depending upon the social, political and psychological mores and norms of the time.

The revolutionary view of psychologist Carl Rogers that in fact the underlying motivational tendency in human beings was positive and trustworthy met – and still meets – with a great deal of scepticism, disbelief and scorn. On many, many occasions Rogers was asked how *anyone* could be so *naive* as to believe that human beings are inherently 'good' when there is clearly so much 'bad' happening in the world around us. He tended to respond to such scepticism, disbelief and scorn in two ways. He acknowledged that *of course* there was the possibility that the human race would eventually destroy itself and even the planet earth in one way or another – for instance, the proliferation of weaponry and environmental damage hardly bodes well. However, he pointed out that there was also the possibility that we would not destroy either ourselves or the planet, and in the meantime he chose to put all of his energy into the potential for positive growth rather than destruction. Secondly, he stated that *of course* therapists encountered many of the more unpleasant and unpalatable aspects of living. Indeed, this very difficulty with human nature is why so many people seek counselling in the first place. However, his experience over and over and over again was that if he could be genuinely respectful and empathically understanding of the apparently negative, aggressive and hostile aspects of human nature and behaviour – if he could be a sensitive companion to such feelings and thoughts without judging, condemning, and trying to control or change them – then *inevitably* he discovered that 'behind' or 'beneath' them are the positive attributes of the actualising tendency. This exactly matches my own experience. In some 30 years as a counsellor I have met with a high number (thousands) of clients who have disclosed anger, hostility, hate, rage and aggression, yet without fail it has transpired that behind their anger lies hurt and pain – and behind their hurt and pain lies a desperate need to simply love and be loved, value and be valued, like and be liked, and so on.

Having said that *given the right conditions* the human organism is essentially trustworthy, co-operative, responsible, creative and forward moving, it is all too apparent that very often people do not encounter conditions that are fully conducive to healthy growth. As was stated earlier on when looking at the notion of incongruence, all too often interpersonal relationships are conditional – there are strings attached. *Unconditional* positive regard ideally has no strings attached, and it is this very unconditional acceptance that, if experienced, tends to reduce feelings of threat and therefore the need for defensiveness (as will be more fully explored when we look at therapeutic process in Chapter 5).

Another link between unconditional positive regard and empathic understanding is that the client-centred therapist *understands* (and accepts) that were *any* human being to have the same history and experience that this particular client has, they would in all likelihood exhibit similar feelings, thoughts and behaviours. There is a kind of 'there but for the grace of fate go I' feel to it. In other words, get the good breaks and chances in life and certain consequences are likely, but get only bad breaks or be deprived of opportunities, and outcomes might be equally predictable – and very *understandable*. Linking congruence *and* unconditional positive regard *and* empathic understanding, let us not forget the importance of therapists offering and being the core conditions *to and for themselves*. If therapists can understand themselves they are likely to be self-accepting, too.

> One way of putting this is that I feel I have become more adequate in letting myself *be* what I *am* . . . It seems to me to have value because the curious paradox is that when I accept myself as I am, I change. I believe that I have learned this from my clients as well as within my own experience – that we cannot change, we cannot move away from what we are, until we thoroughly accept what we are. Then change seems to come about almost unnoticed.
>
> (Rogers 1961: p. 17)

We saw when looking at incongruence how all too often our conditions of worth can be formulated around the values and judgements of significant others, and that these conditions of worth may thwart the positive nature of the actualising tendency. To be congruent, client-centred therapists will have explored and reappraised their conditions of worth, retaining and reintegrating those introjected values that have personal meaning and discarding those introjected values that do not. To be a *client-centred* therapist, unconditional positive regard will have become deeply embedded within the concept of self – not because Carl Rogers said so, but because both the *giving* and the *receiving* of unconditional positive regard have been personally experienced as meaningfully helpful. Unconditional positive regard will be valued from an internal locus of experiential evaluation and be a primary constituent of the therapist's self-concept as an attitudinal way of being that ideally is in complete harmony with the actualising tendency.

If the client-centred practitioner holds an unswerving faith in the primacy and positive nature of the actualising tendency, other consequences follow. Many of these repercussions could be deemed 'political' in nature (and it was only late in his career that Carl Rogers acknowledged the political dimensions of client-centred therapy), such as a belief in the *right* of the individual to *self-determination* or *autonomy*. A belief in the sanctity of the *dignity* of human beings follows, too. If the therapist believes that it is the *therapist* who knows best what is good for the client, then that therapist is blatantly not respectful of the capacity, resources and potential within human beings for autonomy and dignity.

As already stated, Carl Rogers believed one of the most effective ways to communicate unconditional positive regard is to be empathic, as:

> it would appear that for me, as counsellor, to focus my whole attention and effort upon understanding and perceiving as the client perceives and understands, is a striking operational demonstration of the belief I have in the worth and the significance of this individual client. Clearly the most important value which I hold is, as indicated by my attitudes and my verbal behaviour, the client himself. Also the fact that I permit the outcome to rest upon this deep understanding is probably the most vital operational evidence which could be given that I have confidence in the potentiality of the individual for constructive change and development in the direction of a more full and satisfying life. As a seriously disturbed client wrestles with his utter inability to make any choice, or another client struggles with his strong urges to commit suicide, the fact that I enter with deep understanding into the desperate feelings that exist, but do not attempt to take over respons-ibility, is a most meaningful expression of basic confidence in the forward-moving tendencies in the human organism.
>
> We might say, then, that for many therapists functioning from a client-centred orientation, the sincere aim of getting 'within' the attitudes of the client, of entering the client's internal frame of reference, is the most complete implementation which has thus far been formulated, for the central hypothesis of respect for and reliance upon the capacity of the person.
>
> (Rogers 1951: pp. 35–6)

Clients really are worth the therapist's efforts in striving to understand them, and the fact that the 'non-directive' counsellor respects clients' self-direction and self-responsibility is meaningful evidence of the therapist's trust in the inner capacity and resources of clients, who thus perceive (to whatever degree) a very precious and rare respect and trust in themselves.

> If the counsellor maintains this consistently client-centred attitude, and if he occasionally conveys to the client something of his under-standing, then he is doing what he can to give the client the experience of being deeply respected. Here the confused, tentative, almost incoherent thinking of an individual who knows he has been eval-uated as abnormal is really respected by being deemed well worth understanding.
>
> (Rogers 1951: p. 44)

So the client perceives that the therapist holds and lives by an attitude which indicates that the client is worth the effort of striving to understand him or her. Again, this could be reformulated using an 'If–then' approach. *If* person A strives to the utmost to understand person B, *then* person B is likely to perceive how respectful person A is of person B.

> Acceptance does not mean much until it involves understanding. It is only as I *understand* the feelings and thoughts which seem so horrible to you, or so weak, or so sentimental, or so bizarre – it is only as I see them as you see them, and accept them and you, that you feel really free to explore all the hidden nooks and frightening crannies of your inner and often buried experience. This *freedom* is an important condition of the relationship. There is implied here a freedom to explore oneself at both conscious and unconscious levels, as rapidly as one can dare to embark on this dangerous quest. There is also a complete freedom from any type of moral or diagnostic evaluation, since all such evaluations are, I believe, always threatening.
>
> (Rogers 1961: p. 34)

The intertwined nature of unconditional positive regard and empathic understanding comes across very clearly in the following passage written by Carl Rogers in 1980. He states that a consequence of *empathic understanding* is that:

> the recipient feels valued, cared for, accepted as the person that he or she is. It might seem that we have here stepped into another area, and that we are no longer speaking of empathy. But this is not so. It is impossible to accurately sense the perceptual world of another person unless you value that person and his or her world – unless you, in some sense, care. Hence, the message comes through to the recipient that 'this other individual trusts me, thinks I'm worthwhile. Perhaps I *am* worth something. Perhaps *I* could value *myself*. Perhaps I could care for myself'.
>
> (Rogers 1980: pp. 152–3)

Stating that 'The highest expression of empathy is accepting and non-judgmental . . . because it is impossible to be accurately perceptive of another's inner world if you have formed an evaluative opinion of that person', Carl Rogers suggests an experiential way of testing this:

> If you doubt this statement, choose someone you know with whom you deeply disagree and who is, in your judgment, definitely wrong or mistaken. Now try to state that individual's views, beliefs, and feelings so accurately that he or she will agree that you have sensitively and correctly described his or her stance. I predict that nine times out of ten you will fail, because your judgment of the person's views creeps into your description of them.
>
> Consequently, true empathy is always free of any evaluative or diagnostic quality. The recipient perceives this with some surprise: 'If I am not being judged, perhaps I am not so evil or abnormal as I have

thought. Perhaps I don't have to judge myself so harshly.' Thus the possibility of self-acceptance is gradually increased.

(Rogers 1980: p. 154)

Quoting RD Laing (and likening Laing to Buber), Rogers agreed with the notion that 'the sense of identity requires the existence of another by whom one is known' (Laing 1965), and that our very existence is affirmed or confirmed by interaction ('contact') with or being *fully received* by another person. Authentic, respectful, empathic understanding serves to give this 'needed confirmation that one does exist as a separate, valued person with an identity' (Rogers 1980: p. 155).

Having spent so long exploring a necessary and sufficient condition, the comments made by Carl Rogers when he was interviewed for RTE Dublin television in 1985 might seem a little surprising. The interviewer, John Masterson, said to him:

> One of the requirements you place upon yourself is to unconditionally accept and have unconditional positive regard for the person who you are trying to help. That presumably must be very difficult in some cases . . .
>
> (Rogers 1985)

To which Carl Rogers replied:

> No, that's a slight misunderstanding. What I have said is that I am very fortunate in the relationship if that feeling and attitude exists in me. I am very fortunate and the client is very fortunate if I can feel I really accept you fully just as you are.
>
> (Rogers 1985)

This comment was and is extremely liberating for me. For many years my introjected value, my condition of worth, was that experiencing and offering the conditions was both necessary and sufficient, and if I *failed* I would give myself (or be given – maybe by a supervisor or by peers) a hard time. The client-centred conditions had become, at times at least, a stick with which to beat myself, or to be beaten with, or, worse still, as a trainer a stick with which I would beat trainees! Now, some 28 years after first postulating the *necessary and sufficient client-centred conditions* in 1957, here was Carl saying *'No, that's a slight misunderstanding'*. Yet how qualitatively different it is – how uplifting – to feel *fortunate* if I could succeed to some degree as compared with feeling a *failure* if I did not. Rogers continued:

> Sometimes that's very difficult. I held an interview with a young man in South Africa. I didn't know anything about him. It turned out he was an officer in the South African army. Now for me, that meant a real . . . It meant that I stretched my empathic abilities to their very limit, to try to be with him, to try to understand him, to try to be caring toward him. I didn't feel I did too well – and yet I've learned since that interview really changed the course of his life.
>
> (Rogers 1985)

Once again, then, we see how it is that imperfect human beings can be of help to other imperfect human beings – and actually what Rogers said in 1985 was not especially new, as he wrote eight years earlier (in 1978):

> It is not, of course, possible to feel such an unconditional caring all the time. A therapist who is real will often have very different feelings, negative feelings toward the client. Hence it is not to be regarded as a 'should' that the therapist *should* have an unconditional positive regard for the client. It is simply a fact that unless this is a reasonably frequent ingredient in the relationship, constructive client change is less likely.
>
> (Rogers 1978: p. 10)

To think (and experience) in terms of it being *fortunate* if unconditional positive regard frequently exists in the therapeutic relationship feels far more conducive to developing such a respectful attitude than to experience a sense of *failure* if a *condition* is not met.

Now let us turn to empathic understanding, the most effective medium through which clients are able to perceive the deep respect of the therapist for them, this ongoing desire of the therapist to understand, this caring and valuing of the client, and this freedom to explore in a non-judgemental relationship.

Empathy and empathic understanding

> We know from our research that such empathic understanding – understanding with a person, not about him – is such an effective approach that it can bring about major changes in personality.
>
> (Rogers 1961: p. 332)

We have learned that congruence is a *state* and that unconditional positive regard is an *attitude* that is authentic if congruent. The third of the therapist conditions, namely empathic understanding, is a *process* through which congruent unconditional positive regard is most effectively conveyed. Returning again to what Carl Rogers had to say about the relative importance of each of the therapist conditions:

> Then, in my experience, there are other situations in which the empathic way of being has the highest priority. When the other person is hurting, confused, troubled, anxious, alienated, and terrified, or when he or she is doubtful of self-worth, uncertain as to identity, then understanding is called for. The gentle and sensitive companionship of an empathic stance – accompanied, of course, by the other two attitudes – provides illumination and healing. In such situations deep understanding is, I believe, the most precious gift one can give to another.
>
> (Rogers 1975: p. 9)

If the therapist is client-centred, *then* unconditional positive regard and empathic understanding will be deeply held and integrated personal characteristics, especially evident in the therapy hour. *If* the therapist experiences an authentic (that is, congruent) attitude of unconditional positive regard towards a client, *then* the most effective expression of this will be through the process of empathic understanding. This deep understanding is not an understanding *about*, but a delicate sensing of the personal feelings and meanings that reside in another person:

> My belief is that, by extending sensitive empathy to another person, it enables him or her to come forth and gain a better understanding of himself and what direction he is going.
>
> (Rogers and Teich 1992: p. 55)

Empathy and client perception of therapist unconditional positive regard and empathic understanding

Although a counselling relationship can be initiated by the therapist providing the core conditions:

> Unless the attitudes I have been describing have been to some degree communicated to the client, and perceived by him, they do not exist in his perceptual world and thus cannot be effective. Consequently it is necessary to add one more condition to the equation . . . It is that when the client perceives, to a minimal degree, the genuineness of the counselor and the acceptance and empathy which the counselor experiences for him, then development in personality and change in behavior are predicted.
>
> (Rogers and Stevens 1967: p. 96)

Two people are in contact (or psychological contact, if preferred), each making a perceived difference in the experiential (or perceptual, or phenomenological) world of the other. We have already seen that:

> In a deeply defended person . . . change is difficult to bring about. Change tends to occur more in the person who is already somewhat open-minded and searching in his approach to life.
>
> (Rogers and Evans 1975: p. 73)

Thus clients entering therapy are likely to be *seekers* – they will be in stage two of the process. The therapist is congruent in the relationship and the client is incongruent, being vulnerable or anxious. The therapist experiences unconditional positive regard towards and engages in a process of empathic understanding of the client. The notion of reciprocal empathy links with client perception of the therapist's empathy. Rogers said:

> It seems to me that the moment where persons are most likely to change, or I even think of it as the moments in which people *do* change, are the moments in which perhaps the relationship is experienced the same on both sides.
>
> (Rogers 1989: p. 53)

The therapist's perception of the client is motivated by an authentic desire to continually respect and understand that client's world from within the client's internal frame of reference. While therapists 'perception check' their sensing of clients' feelings and personal meanings, the notion of reciprocal empathy indicates that, to some degree, therapists rely on the capacity of their client to empathise with and understand their therapist's attempts to empathically under-stand that client. As Rogers wrote when reviewing various studies:

> it is the attitudes and feelings of the therapist, rather than his theoretical orientation, which are important. His procedures and techniques are less important than his attitudes. It is also worth noting that it is the way in which his attitudes and procedures are *perceived* which makes a crucial difference to the client, and that it is this perception which is crucial.
>
> (Rogers 1961: p. 44)

Whether through the therapist's ongoing desire to understand or via reciprocated empathy, for a therapeutic relationship and engagement in a therapeutic process to occur, the authentic unconditional positive regard and empathic understand-ing of the therapist must be perceived by the client *at least to a minimal degree* (or in terms of the therapist striving to communicate respect and empathy, then *at least to a minimal degree* such communication needs to be achieved):

> We know that if the therapist holds within himself attitudes of deep respect and full acceptance for this client as he is, and similar attitudes toward the client's potentialities for dealing with himself and his situations; if these attitudes are suffused with a sufficient warmth, which transforms them into the most profound type of liking or affection for the core of the person; and if a level of communication is reached so that the client can begin to perceive that the therapist understands the feelings he is experiencing and accepts them at the full depth of that understanding, then we may be sure that the process is already initiated.
>
> (Rogers 1961: pp. 74–5)

What does '*at least to a minimal degree*' actually *mean*? Does it mean that if during a therapy session a therapist communicates, say, 20 times, and three or four of those communications could be deemed authentically respectful and empathic, then the condition of *at least to a minimal degree* has been met (despite 16 or 17 communications *not* being respectful or empathic)? Does it mean that if the therapist is authentically respectful and empathic for 5 minutes out of 50 this condition has been met? Does it mean that if every therapist communication is characterised by *low* levels of authentic unconditional positive regard and empathic understanding, then at least to a minimal degree the sixth condition has been achieved? Carl Rogers wrote that:

> This struggle to achieve the client's internal frame of reference, to gain the center of his own perceptual field and see with him as perceiver, is rather closely analogous to some of the Gestalt phenomena. Just as, by active concentration, one can suddenly see the diagram in the psych-ology text as representing a descending rather than an ascending stairway or can perceive two faces instead of a candlestick, so by active effort the counselor can put himself into the client's frame of reference. But just as in the case of the visual perception, the figure occasionally changes, so the counselor may at times find himself standing outside the client's frame of reference and looking as an

external perceiver at the client. This almost invariably happens, for example, during a long pause or silence on the client's part. The counselor may gain a few clues which permit an accurate empathy, but to some extent he is forced to view the client from an observer's point of view, and can only actively assume the client's perceptual field when some type of expression again begins.

(Rogers 1951: p. 32)

There are nearly always 'some clues' that the therapist can absorb or sense. Equally, while the therapist might *constantly strive* to empathically understand, it is extremely unlikely that deep empathic understanding will be experienced as *constant*. There may be some clues, too, as to how training in client-centred therapy helps to bring about increased empathy. When comparing types of counsellor communications in written papers before and after training, even back in 1951 Carl Rogers found that there was increased 'reflection' (from around 50% to around 85%), and decreased interpretation (from approximately 19% to around 11%). Support, and moralising were reduced to zero (from around 8% and 5% respectively), and diagnosing fell from about 18% to 3%. Studying counselling practice produced similar results. 'Reflection' increased (from around 11% to 59%), as did information giving (from 2.5% to 3.9%) and 'innocuous' communications such as acceptance or silence (from around 5% to 11%). There was reduced interpretation (from 22% to 15%), support (from 15% to 5%), 'oughtness' (from 20% to 3%), information seeking (from 16% to 2%) and personal opinion (from 9% to 1%) (Rogers 1951: p. 455).

Degrees of empathy

The notion of low, intermediate and high levels of empathy was briefly introduced in Chapter 1. In summary:

At a relatively low level of empathic sensitivity the therapist responds with clarity only to the patient's most obvious feelings. At an intermediate level, the therapist usually responds accurately to the client's more obvious feelings and occasionally recognizes some that are less apparent, but in the process of tentative probing, he may anticipate feelings which are not current or may misinterpret the present feelings. At a higher level, the therapist is aware of many feelings and experiences which are not so evident, but his lack of complete understanding is shown by the slightly inaccurate nature of his deeper responses . . . At a very high level of empathic understanding, the therapist's responses move, with sensitivity and accuracy, into feelings and experiences that are only hinted at by the client.

It is this sensitive and accurate grasp and communication of the patient's inner world that facilitates the patient's self-exploration and consequent personality growth.

(Rogers and Truax 1967: p. 106)

Yet further clues about degrees of empathic understanding might be gained from the work of Barrett-Lennard (quoted by Carl Rogers) who developed a Relationship Inventory (Barrett-Lennard 1959) that in part tried to measure the degree to which clients felt empathically understood. Thus a scale from high to low empathy looked like this:

- He appreciates what my experience feels like to *me*.
- He tries to see things through my eyes.
- Sometimes he thinks that I feel a certain way because he feels that way.
- He understands what I say from a detached, objective point of view.
- He understands my words but not the way I feel.

Over the years, a variety of writers from a range of different orientations have come up with a variety of empathy 'rating scales' or other strategies for evaluating the degree of empathy (or empathic understanding) deemed to be present in a (therapeutic) relationship. While in person-centred counsellor training there may well be an across-the-board agreement that developing empathy is a fundamental aspect of the learning, there would appear to be little or no agreement on measuring or evaluating the *degree* of empathy necessary as evidence of practice good enough to merit the award of a diploma, despite the UK Government's focus on 'benchmarking'. It is also true to say that, over the years, there has been some resistance to empathy 'rating scales' in person-centred circles. For instance, some evaluation mechanisms have been perceived as overly mechanistic – 'add 0.5 to stage three if a later element is present', 'subtract 0.25 if an earlier element is missing', and so on.

However, formulating *some* kind of structure for exploring the degree of empathy that might (or might not) be present in counselling relationships might still be helpful for two main reasons. First, therapists in the UK (and maybe this is especially true of 'person-centred' counsellors or those in existential and 'humanistic' schools) have tended to be rather 'anti-evaluation' because such monitoring is reminiscent of 'Big Brother'-type meddling. Yet as therapists perhaps we *should* be accountable – to our clients, to ourselves, and to our profession (and to our employer, if we have one). Secondly, any activity that has the potential to develop a client-centred therapeutic way of being is worth engaging in. Ongoing monitoring of the degree to which therapists are able both to experience empathy and to communicate their sensing of client feelings and meanings could be valuable in terms of personal and professional development. Here, then, is an attempt to define some of the significant characteristics of empathic understanding (this time from low to high) (Vincent 2002c):

- Level A: The therapist communicates some *understanding* of what the client is experiencing in the moment, if only in a somewhat diluted way.
- Level B: The therapist communicates some sensing of what the client is *feeling* in the here and now, if only in a somewhat diluted way.
- Level C: The therapist communicates some sensing of what the client's present experiencing *means* to the client, if only in a somewhat diluted way.
- Level D: The therapist communicates some *understanding* of what the client is experiencing in the moment, at approximately the same intensity as the client's disclosure.
- Level E: The therapist communicates some sensing of what the client is *feeling* in the here and now, at approximately the same intensity as the client's disclosure.

- Level F: The therapist communicates some sensing of what the client's present experiencing *means* to the client, at approximately the same intensity as the client's disclosure.
- Level G: The therapist communicates some sensing of what the client is *feeling* in the moment, and a degree of *understanding* why the client feels as she does, if only in a somewhat diluted way.
- Level H: The therapist communicates some sensing of what the client is *feeling* in the here and now, some *understanding* of why the client feels as she does, and a degree of sensing what this experiencing *means* to the client, if only in a somewhat diluted way.
- Level I: The therapist communicates some sensing of what the client is *feeling* in the moment, and a degree of *understanding* why the client feels as she does, at approximately the same intensity as the client's disclosure.
- Level J: The therapist communicates some sensing of what the client is *feeling* in the here and now, some *understanding* of why the client feels as she does, and a degree of sensing what this experiencing *means* to the client, at approximately the same intensity as the client's disclosure.
- Level K: The therapist communicates some sensing of here-and-now client *feelings* at an intensity similar to the client's disclosure, and feelings of which the client seems only dimly aware.
- Level L: The therapist communicates some sensing of what the client is *feeling* in the here and now, some *understanding* of why the client feels as she does, and a degree of sensing what this experiencing *means* to the client, at approximately the same intensity as the client's disclosure, together with sensing feelings and meanings of which the client seems only dimly aware.

Anything presented as a hierarchy carries with it the danger that, to give an example, *empathy level L* is far more desirable than *empathy level A* – and the whole picture isn't as clear as that. For instance, there can be a tendency (especially within person-centred circles) to value feelings ('gut stuff') above thoughts ('head stuff'). Yet any valuing of one aspect of empathic understanding above another hardly sits comfortably with *unconditional* positive regard of whatever a client is experiencing from moment to moment. Suppose that in a first session with a client I notice upon reflection that many of my communications are characteristic of empathy level A. Does this mean that I have to give myself a hard time and beat myself up? No, it doesn't have to mean that I must come down really heavily on myself. It could be, for instance, that if I replay the tape inserting alternative communications at *empathy level L*, I realise that to have done so at the time would have been inappropriate and insensitive in the extreme to what the client was experiencing in that moment. Had I communicated at empathy level L throughout, maybe my main intent would have been to demonstrate my own cleverness or something – certainly not client-centred!

Something akin to this formulation of degrees of empathic understanding might be of use to (trainee) therapists when analysing a tape-recorded client session. The tape can be paused at any point and the therapist's communication can then be explored, looking at the degree to which empathy was experienced, the extent to which empathic understanding was communicated, the links between the levels of experienced and communicated empathy and where the client and therapist are in terms of therapeutic process, and the level, appropriateness and sensitivity of each and every spoken word.

In the previous example, it was stated that a constant striving for *level L* empathic understanding in a first session might be more to do with a therapist needing to prove their own cleverness than with demonstrating respect for and sensitivity to the client. On the other hand, if a therapist realises upon reflection that only understanding (*level A*) was communicated when feelings and meanings were evident, then there is an opportunity to explore why this might have been, and why at the time the counsellor was unable to experience and offer, say, *level C* empathy. Again, let this format come with a health warning. If this kind of reflecting on practice becomes too mechanistic, the essence of the I–thou relationship could well be lost.

Carl Rogers seemed keen to take a step back from rating each and every therapist communication on empathy scales. Perhaps like his daughter Natalie he feared that a microscopic obsession with detail ran the risk of losing the essence of the I–thou relationship – and Rogers definitely feared (as we have already seen) that a possible consequence of focusing too minutely on counsellor responses could lead to a proliferation of cold, wooden techniques and skills training. Perhaps it might make sense, then, to transpose something that he wrote when asked how long counsellor training should be. He said:

> some training is better than none, more training is better than some.
> (Rogers 1951: p. 442)

Our answer, then, to the question 'What does *at least to a minimal degree* actually mean?' could be:

- *Some unconditional positive regard is better than none.*
- *More unconditional positive regard is better than some.*

and

- *Some empathic understanding is better than none.*
- *More empathic understanding is better than some.*

Finally, Rogers wrote:

> And with clients in therapy, I am often impressed with the fact that even a minimal amount of empathic understanding – a bumbling and faulty attempt to catch the confused complexity of the client's meaning – is helpful, though there is no doubt that it is most helpful when I can see and formulate clearly the meanings in his experiencing which for him have been unclear and tangled.
> (Rogers 1961: pp. 53–4)

In Chapter 5 we shall explore the impact of some empathy being better than none and more being better than some in relation to client-centred therapeutic process. The journey of untangling begins . . .

Summary

Contact

Carl Rogers and his colleagues learned that a describable, sequential and orderly process, similar for all clients, was a predictable consequence of incongruent clients coming into contact (that is, being in a relationship within which each person is aware of the other) with a therapist for whom authentic respect and empathy were key personal traits. When the therapist is client-centred and the client is incongruent and contact has been established:

> then we may be sure that the process is already initiated.
>
> (Rogers 1961: pp. 74–5)

Client incongruence

We have seen that Carl Rogers believed it was essential for therapists to understand the intellectual context of therapy, and this includes an in-depth understanding of the concepts behind all of the necessary and sufficient conditions for personality change, including the nature of human beings and how they experience, and a concept of the self – if only because it is so relevant to clients (and this is about *client*-centred therapy). Incongruence, wrote Carl Rogers:

> results when the individual's experience is quite discrepant from the way he has organized himself.
>
> (Rogers and Evans 1975: pp. 19–20)

The conditions of worth embedded in a client's self-concept may well have served to thwart his or her actualising tendency.

Therapist congruence

Congruence is a construct composed of five main elements, namely congruence of self and experience, openness to experience, psychological adjustment, extensionality and maturity.

> It means that he is *being* himself, not denying himself. No one fully achieves this condition, yet the more the therapist is able to listen acceptantly to what is going on within himself, and the more he is able to be the complexity of his feelings without fear, the higher the degree of his congruence.
>
> (Rogers and Stevens 1967: pp. 90–1)

However, it is crucial to understand that:

> Being real does not involve us doing anything we want to do; it means a disciplined approach.
>
> (Rogers and Russell 2002: p. 284)

Therapy cannot be considered to be client-centred if therapist congruence does not as the primary feature include deeply integrated and experienced respect and empathy. As this too is so crucial, let us again read that:

For therapy to occur the wholeness of the therapist in the relationship is primary, but a part of the congruence of the therapist must be the experience of unconditional positive regard and the experience of empathic understanding.

(Rogers 1959: p. 215)

Therapist unconditional positive regard

Unconditional positive regard is about valuing a person without judging that person as good or bad, or as more or less worthy of respect:

Unconditional positive regard, when communicated by the therapist, serves to provide the nonthreatening context in which the client can explore and experience the most deeply shrouded elements of his inner self. The therapist is neither paternalistic, nor sentimental, nor superficially social and agreeable. But his deep caring is a necessary ingredient of the 'safe' context in which the client can come to explore himself and share deeply with another human being.

(Rogers 1989: p. 14)

Therapist empathic understanding

Carl wrote that:

to enter deeply with this man into his confused struggle for selfhood is perhaps the best implementation we now know for indicating the meaning of our basic hypothesis that the individual represents a process which is deeply worthy of respect, both as he is and with regard to his potentialities.

(Rogers 1951: p. 45)

Entering deeply, sensitively and delicately into a client's world means sensing their feelings and personal meanings as if you were that client, yet having a strong enough sense of your own selfhood to ensure that you remain a companion and do not get lost in the other's world.

The client perceives . . .

The client-centred therapist has *presence* in the relationship – so much so that nothing other than the client's world of feelings and meanings matters very much to the therapist during the client's time. There is a very real sense of two people being deeply connected (or at least the client senses that the therapist is striving towards a profound engagement). In striving to enter fully the private world of another individual, the therapist to some degree relies upon the client to empathise with and understand this effort – hence the notion of reciprocal empathy.

So the client-centred therapist strives to be in a *state* of *congruence* when with clients, a state that incorporates an authentic (because it is congruent), deeply held *attitude* of *unconditional positive regard* that is perceived by clients through a *process* of *empathic understanding*.

If
a person is incongruent,
then
they might seek counselling.

If
the therapist is congruent,
then
unconditional positive regard will, in harmony with the actualising tendency, be deeply embedded and integrated within the therapist's self-concept.

If
the therapist is congruently respectful,
then
the client will perceive this through the process of being empathically understood by the therapist.

If
the client receives congruent unconditional positive regard and empathic understanding,
then
a therapeutic process will unfold.

In other words,

If
the therapist can
be
the core conditions,
then
the client will
do
the rest.

Empathic understanding and therapeutic process

Therapist be, client do

Carl Rogers wrote of empathy:

> We know from our research that such empathic understanding –
> understanding *with* a person, not *about* him – is such an effective
> approach that it can bring about major changes in personality.
>
> (Rogers 1961: p. 332)

Having looked earlier at the notion of two people coming into (at least minimal)
contact, and how a therapeutic *relationship* might be established in which the client
feels *received*, we can now begin to fathom what these 'major changes in
personality' might be and how they might come about. Rogers wrote that
client-centred therapeutic process is:

> [a] unique and dynamic experience, different for each individual, yet
> exhibiting a lawfulness and order which is astonishing in its generality.
>
> (Rogers 1961: p. 74)

Carl became increasingly disinterested in questions such as 'Does client-centred
therapy *apply* to this, that or the other, and will it *cure* these ailments?'. While
acknowledging that, for some individuals, hospitalisation, drugs or other medical
aid might well be appropriate, he wrote:

> client-centered therapy is very widely applicable – indeed in one sense
> it is applicable to all people. An atmosphere of acceptance and respect,
> of deep understanding, is a good climate for personal growth . . . This
> does *not* mean that it will *cure* every psychological condition, and
> indeed the concept of cure is quite foreign to the approach . . . Yet a
> psychological climate which the individual can use for deeper self-
> understanding, for a reorganization of self in the direction of more
> realistic integration, for the development of more comfortable and
> mature ways of behaving – this is not an opportunity which is of use
> for some groups and not for others. It would appear rather to be a point
> of view which might in basic ways be applicable to all individuals, even
> though it might not resolve all the problems or provide all the help
> which a particular individual needs.
>
> (Rogers 1951: p. 230)

While Rogers was not in any way opposed to legitimate and reasonable
questioning of client-centred therapy, he also proposed that the asking of such
questions was akin to enquiring whether gamma rays would be an appropriate

application or cure for chilblains! It is perhaps interesting to note that the 'Ah yes, but does this type of therapy apply to or cure A, B and C through to X, Y and Z?' type enquiry is only rarely encountered as a critique of approaches *other* than client-centred therapy, when in fact there is little or no evidence whatsoever to suggest that client-centred therapy (or person-centred counselling) is any less effective than any other approach. Indeed, there is a growing body of national and international evidence (e.g. Friedli *et al.* 1977: pp. 1662–5; King *et al.* 2000: pp. 1383–8) that in fact client-centred therapy is the most effective approach.

In Southampton Primary Care Trust, from 2003 to 2004, client-centred therapy proved to be the most effective therapeutic approach, with over 90% of patients showing improvement (as measured by CORE, Clinical Outcomes in Routine Evaluation), less than 8% showing no change, and 1% showing deterioration. Gestalt and transactional analysis faired similarly. Psychodynamic, structured/brief and integrative approaches all showed between 70% and 80% improvement, with 10–20% of patients (approximately) showing no change and with 0–10% showing deterioration. Cognitive–behavioural therapy showed less than 70% improvement, with 30% of patients showing no change, and no patient showing deterioration (Vincent 2004).

Nevertheless, Carl Rogers consistently remained disinterested in comparing client-centred with other approaches, preferring instead to write and speak of his own view: 'I'll just speak about what you call my end of it' (Rogers and Evans 1975: p. 116) and 'rather than try to comment on such approaches . . . I'd rather say something about my own view' (Rogers and Evans 1975: p. 5). Rather than engage in such wrangling, he instead approached those issues by stating that client-centred therapy is a describable *process*, with a *core of sequential orderly events* that tend to be present *for all* clients.

> The practice of person-centred therapy dramatizes its differences from most other orientations. Therapy begins immediately; with the therapist trying to understand the client's world in whatever way the client wishes to share it.
>
> (Rogers and Raskin 1989: p. 172)

While some counsellors may begin by greeting clients and then launching into taking case histories, or meeting some other administrative, bureaucratic, 'professional' or 'therapeutic' needs, the client-centred therapist *begins immediately* by authentically respecting and striving to understand. Thus if clients look anxious and seem uncertain where to begin, client-centred therapists are likely to voice something of their sensing of where clients are, in the moment. So *therapy begins immediately* - and provided that the necessary and sufficient conditions exist, a process will unfold that has predictable outcomes. *If* the necessary and sufficient conditions (A) are met, *then* a therapeutic process (B) ensues, and *if* a therapeutic relationship (B) exists over time, *then* there are predictable outcomes (C) in terms of personality change. What, then, is the process, and what outcomes can be predicted?

Process models

> It has been the experience of many, counselors and clients alike, that when the counselor has adopted in a genuine way the function which

he understands to be characteristic of a client-centered counselor, the client tends to have a vital and releasing experience which has many similarities from one client to another.

(Rogers 1951: p. 49)

How can we explore and understand the process of client-centred therapy? Carl Rogers wrote that:

> Therapy has always been interesting to me as a process of change . . . I realize I'm a person who is greatly interested in process, and I don't know quite how to put this, but I know part of my concern about philosophy of science grew out of the fact that there is no objective way of testing process. You have to slice the process and take a cross-section of it at point *A* and point *B* and see the difference. That's the process. But there is no such thing as an objective study of a long-itudinal changing process; and that's just an intriguing aspect about science – that . . . you can prove that change takes place; you can prove the nature of that change, but you don't study the process as it occurs. You study it by taking samples at different points and investigating those.

(Rogers and Russell 2002: p. 270)

Several 'models' of therapeutic process can be found within the writings of Carl Rogers, mostly consisting of or constructed around these 'slices' or cross-sections into the process, and hence there is a marked tendency to present process as a sequence of stages or phases. The earliest model of non-directive process was composed of just three phases, namely *release, insight,* and *positive action* based on insight:

> In the earliest description of client-centered therapy, I pictured the process as composed primarily of three steps . . . first, in the release of expression, the release of personal feelings . . . Following this emotional catharsis, insight tended to develop into the origin and nature of the difficulties being experienced by the client. Such insight was followed by the making of positive choices and decisions in regard to the problem elements of the client's life – an emotional re-education involved in the practice of applying the newly gained insights in reality.

(Rogers 1989: p. 23)

However, Carl soon learned from the data gained through research that greater emphasis needed to be placed on looking into the notion of the client's self and how clients experienced processes of disorganisation and reintegration within the self.

> I think those concepts were the first rather simple attempt to understand what was going on. I suppose, in looking back on them, I feel they were oversimplified but accurate so far as they went. That release of pent-up feelings is important – there's much more to it than that:

> the development of insight is important, and I don't feel therapy is
> complete unless it evolves into some sort of positive action.
>
> (Rogers and Russell 2002: p. 246)

In 1951, Rogers published his findings on how *clients* experienced the process. It seems in keeping with client-centred philosophy that given the primacy of the belief and trust in the dignity, resources and rights of clients (as compared with the authority and knowledge of therapies or therapists), *clients* are placed at the heart of describing and understanding how therapy is experienced. Remember that it was through listening to and striving to understand clients that Rogers learned much of what became formulated as client-centred therapy and the person-centred approach – it could be said that *his clients taught Carl Rogers all that he knew* (or at least much of what he came to know). A five-stage model emerged from researching what clients had to report about their therapy. They tended to experience:

1 responsibility
2 the discovery of denied attitudes
3 a reorganising of the self
4 progress
5 ending.

Later, in 1961, a seven-stage model was developed that is included here because it is still used by many programmes in the UK as the 'main' training resource. People in *stage 1* are unlikely to refer themselves for therapy, as they are remote from their experience and in a 'fixed' state of being. They are unwilling to communicate in personal depth (instead referring only to external factors), and their inner communications are also significantly blocked, so both feelings and meanings are neither recognised nor owned. Relational depth is viewed as dangerous and there is no desire to grow, as basically people at this stage do not see themselves as having a problem.

It is noteworthy that throughout this model of process (other than between stages 6 and 7) Rogers saw it as essential that *the client must experience being fully received in one stage prior to moving into the next.* Again we see the *'If–then'* nature of client-centred theory. *If* clients experience themselves as fully received in one stage, *then* they can move into the next. If clients do feel fully received in stage 1, *stage 2* involves a slight increase in disclosure, although issues are still viewed as external to the self. Feelings are disowned and are sometimes seen as belonging to the past, and there is little sense of responsibility for them. The organisation of the self is still rigid or fixed and seen as a static fact. Even if contradictory feelings and meanings are verbalised, there is no awareness of their contradictory nature. *If the client feels fully received* in stage 2, then there is a movement in *stage 3* towards talking about the self, although the self is still viewed as an object and often only seen through the way in which others view that self. Feelings and meanings may be described, but they are not felt as present in the here and now and they are mostly unacceptable, being seen as somehow 'bad', shameful or embarrassing. There is still a sense of remoteness from experiencing, although some feelings are spoken of and there may be some recognition of personal constructs within the self, albeit still as objects. There is slightly less generalising and some recognition of contradictions, although any choices that the client has made are usually seen as inadequate. If the client feels fully received in stage 3, then they can move into stages 4 and 5, which according to Carl Rogers:

> constitute much of psychotherapy as we know it.
>
> (Rogers 1961: p. 139)

When clients feel that they have been welcomed, received, and understood and accepted just as they are, then in *stage 4* personal constructs tend to become slightly less rigid and feelings begin to flow more readily:

> The client describes more intense feelings of the 'not-now-present' variety. Feelings are described as objects in the present. Occasionally feelings are expressed as in the present, sometimes breaking through almost against the client's wishes. There is a tendency toward experiencing feelings in the immediate present, and there is distrust and fear of this possibility. There is little open acceptance of feelings, though some acceptance is exhibited. Experiencing is less bound by the structure of the past, is less remote, and may occasionally occur with little postponement. There is a loosening of the way experience is construed. There are some discoveries of personal constructs; there is the definite recognition of these as constructs; and there is a beginning questioning of their validity. There is an increased differentiation of feelings, constructs, personal meanings, with some tendency toward seeking exactness of symbolization. There is a realization of concern about contradictions and incongruences between experience and self. There are feelings of self-responsibility in problems, though such feelings vacillate. Though a close relationship still feels dangerous, the client risks himself, relating to some small extent on a feeling basis.
>
> (Rogers 1961: pp. 137–8)

Once clients feel fully received in stage 4, yet further processing is set in motion, characterised in *stage 5* by freely expressed and experienced current feelings, despite these often being accompanied by feelings of distrust and fear, and hence often surprise. However, there is an increasing desire to both own and be such feelings, as personal constructs move toward reduced fixity and so can be questioned and explored. Clients exhibit fewer generalisations and strive to be more precise when differentiating between feelings and personal meanings, and begin to face their incongruence and contradictions. As greater acceptance of self-responsibility accrues, so there are more meaningful internal dialogues.

At this point, Rogers stepped aside from his narrative to clarify that this is not necessarily a smooth, even process – clients might 'take two steps forward, one step back', and can journey back to previous stages as new disclosures occur. The idea is more of a general trend and movement towards greater self-actualisation which, if the client feels fully received in stage 5, enters *stage 6*. Carl stated that this stage was frequently dramatic and very distinctive:

> A feeling which has previously been 'stuck', has been inhibited in its process quality, is experienced with immediacy now. A feeling flows to its full result. A present feeling is directly experienced with immediacy and richness. This immediacy of experiencing, and the feeling which constitutes its content, are accepted. This is something which is not

something to be denied, feared, struggled against. There is a quality of living subjectively in the experience, not feeling about it. Self as an object tends to disappear. Experiencing, at this stage, takes on a real process quality. Another characteristic of this stage of the process is the physiological loosening which accompanies it. The incongruence between experience and awareness is vividly experienced as it disappears into congruence. The relevant personal construct is dissolved in this experiencing moment, and the client feels cut loose from his previously stabilized framework. The moment of full experiencing becomes a clear and definite referent. Differentiation of experiencing is sharp and basic. In this stage, there are no longer 'problems', external or internal. The client is living, subjectively, a phase of his problem. It is not an object.

(Rogers 1961: pp. 145–50)

Carl also believed that there was almost an *irreversibility* about such moments of immediacy of experience that are fully accepted. As there is a sense of the outcomes of this process by now being irreversible, it is no longer so necessary (although it is still very helpful) for the client to feel fully received prior to entering *stage 7*, in which experiencing of new feelings is both rich and immediate, both inside and outside of counselling. Clients access, own and directly trust their inner experiencing, and are more *process* than *object* beings, becoming more here-and-now oriented. As there is less need for defensive denial or distortion, self-configurations may be reformulated and loosely held, in that they will be constantly checked against ongoing experiencing:

He has changed, but what seems most significant, he has become an integrated process of changingness.

(Rogers 1961: p. 158)

In summary, then, within this model, clients were deemed to experience a 'loosening' of feeling, changes in their manner of experiencing, shifts from incongruence to congruence, changes in the manner and extent to which they communicated the self in a receptive climate, a 'loosening' of the 'cognitive maps' of experience, changes in their relationship to 'their problems', and changes in their manner of relating.

A ten-point overview (that included much of the personality theory covered in Chapter 4 of this book) of what *clients* bring to *client*-centred therapeutic process was included in Carl's 1959 paper entitled 'A theory of therapy, personality, and interpersonal relationships, as developed in the client-centered framework'. This charted the characteristics of the human infant, the development of self, the development of need for positive regard, the development of need for self-regard, the development of conditions of worth, the development of incongruence between self and experience, the development of discrepancies in behaviour, experiences of threat and the process of defence, the process of breakdown and disorganisation, and the process of reintegration. It is the last two, namely the *process of breakdown and disorganisation* and the *process of reintegration*, that are especially relevant once a client has entered therapy. In the same paper, Carl posited the characteristics of a *deteriorating* relationship (with the self and others) and the process whereby relationships (again, with the self and others) *improve*.

With both *reintegration* and the process of an *improving* relationship, client experiencing of the client-centred *therapist* conditions (authentic respect and empathy) are at the core. Having quoted the necessary and sufficient conditions for therapeutic process, Rogers stated that when they were in place a process with 12 characteristic steps would unfold.

In step 1, clients become increasingly expressive (verbally, paraverbally and non-verbally). In *step 2*, such expressions move towards having more reference to the self (rather than to others or to situations). In *step 3* there is increasingly accurate symbolisation of experience, characterised by greater awareness of the differences between feelings and perceptions, and between self, others and contextual factors – and there is greater awareness of the interplay between all of the preceding steps. In *step 4* clients become more aware of incongruence between their self-concepts and their experience. In *step 5*, the threat of such incongruence is experienced.

(At this point in the process, Carl Rogers highlights therapist unconditional positive regard for clients as a key factor, stating that clients are only able to experience the threat that awareness of their incongruence brings because the therapist is as accepting and respectful of incongruence as of congruence, and as accepting of anxiety as of being anxiety free.)

In *step 6*, clients are now able to be fully aware of and experience feelings that have up until now been either denied or distorted. In *step 7* there follows a process of reorganising the self-concept in order to include previously denied or distorted experiences. In *step 8* this ongoing reorganising of the self-concept produces more and more congruence between self and experience, so experience that had up until now been too threatening to symbolise accurately in awareness can now be incorporated.

(A further consequence of *step 8* is that fewer new or ongoing experiences will be perceived as threatening, and hence there will be less denial or distortion of perceptions, and therefore less need to be defensive.)

In *step 9*, as a result, the client is more open to experiencing the unconditional positive regard of the therapist without attendant feelings of threat. In *step 10*, clients begin to feel a sense of unconditional positive *self*-regard. In *step 11*, clients move towards experiencing themselves as the primary locus of evaluation. In *step 12*, organismic valuing becomes more prominent as valuing based on a reaction to conditions of worth recedes.

Having offered this 12-step model of therapeutic process, Carl Rogers then stated that he was in no doubt that students would be puzzled by the absence of any statements about the 'mechanisms' (skills, techniques or procedures) that bring such processes about. He again pointed us to the *'If–then'* nature of his theory – *if* these conditions are present, *then* these processes are a natural and understandable (and predictable) consequence. In experiential terms, *if* you drop a pencil, *then* it will fall to the floor. You might not fully understand the theory of gravity or other relevant factors, yet you can say with some certainty that *if* the condition of standing on the planet earth is met, *then* when you let go of the pencil it will drop – not stay where it is, float off sideways or shoot upwards. In the early years of developing client-centred therapy, Rogers tended to write in terms of *propositions, hypotheses* and *speculation*. However, subsequent research has tended to strongly support, corroborate and validate client-centred beliefs, theory and practices.

In addition to stating that client-centred therapy *begins immediately*, Carl Rogers also wrote that to begin with the process must be *initiated*, and that *therapist attitude* is of primary importance – that client-centred therapists hold a deep respect *for* and full acceptance *of* clients *as they are in the here and now*. The client-centred therapist also believes fundamentally in clients having the innate potentialities for 'dealing' or coping with themselves and their situations. Rogers wrote that:

> If these attitudes are suffused with a sufficient warmth, which transforms them into the most profound type of liking or affection for the core of the person; and if a level of communication is reached so that the client can begin to perceive that the therapist understands the feelings [the client] is experiencing and accepts [the client] at the full depth of that understanding, then we may be sure that the process is already initiated.
>
> (Rogers 1961: pp. 74–5)

Rather than enquire as to whether or not client-centred therapeutic process served specific ends, Rogers was more inclined to research into the *nature* of this process, looking for its inherent characteristics and what direction or directions it tends to take, and what (if any) the natural end-points of the process might be. He wrote:

> *I enjoy the discovering of order in experience*. It seems inevitable that I seek for the meaning or the orderliness . . . Thus I have come to see both scientific research and the process of theory construction as being aimed toward the inward ordering of significant experience . . . So I have come to recognize that the reason I devote myself to research, and to the building of theory, is to satisfy a need for perceiving order and meaning, a subjective need which exists in me.
>
> (Rogers 1961: pp. 74–5)

In his book entitled *Client-Centred Therapy* (Rogers 1951), Carl had already attempted to gain understanding of the fundamental processes and to honestly and openly describe them. He was clear that he was keen to avoid 'warping' his ideas about process in order that they might somehow fit with or 'prove' any preconceived theories or clinical needs. Carl noted that there *were* certain characteristics of client movement, such as an increase in insightful statements, an increase in maturity of reported behaviour, an increase in positive attitude as therapy progresses, a change in perception of and acceptance of the self, the incorporation of previously denied experience into the self-structure, and a shift in the locus of evaluation from outside to inside the self. In other words, as therapy proceeds *the therapeutic relationship changes, personality structure changes*, as does *behaviour* and the *physiological condition* of the client. Carl wrote that even though such reflections upon therapeutic process might prove to be faulty descriptions, they were nevertheless part of an authentic attempt to understand what happens when clients and counsellors engage in a client-centred therapeutic experience.

Pride of place here is given to the five-stage model that Carl presented in 1961, first as it, too, is based on how *clients* reported their experience of therapy, and second, because it is my own favourite, mainly because it feels more *personal*. The five stages are as follows: *Stage 1*, experiencing of the potential self; *Stage 2*, the full experiencing of an affectional relationship; *Stage 3*, the liking of one's self; *Stage 4*, the discovery that the core of personality is positive; and *Stage 5* being one's organism, one's experience.

Experiencing of the potential self

Experiencing of the potential self could more accurately be described as the *awareness of experiencing* or even the *'experiencing of experience'*. In client-centred therapy, given the relative absence of implied or actual threat from the counsellor, clients could explore experiencing *as they actually experienced it*, and without any strong need to *deny* or *distort* that experiencing in an attempt to 'fit' it into the existing concept of self. Thus if as a client I do not feel too threatened by my therapist, *I can be me*, in the here and now – I can experience at different levels *who I am* and *how I am* being me. As much of such experiencing may well represent an extreme contradiction to the client's existing concept of self, there is often a theme along the lines of 'I cannot deny that this is how I am, yet it feels very at odds with who I am', and very often therapists hear phrases from clients such as 'It was out of character' or 'I was beside myself with . . .' or 'It's not like me at all', 'I don't know what came over me', and so on. Such expressions may be part of a process that could be formulated along the lines of 'I am experiencing a me that feels quite different from any part of my experience to date', and this moves tentatively towards 'Well, maybe there are quite a few different selves within me – or at least I have within me rather more contradictions or differences than I had realised', and this in turn moves towards 'I felt certain that it was not possible for me to *be* all of my experiences or all of my selves, because some of those experiences and some of those selves just seemed too at odds with one another – yet I am beginning to think that, just maybe, I can be all of my selves and all of my experiencing'. In other words, the client moves *away from* being a conglomeration of disparate, separate and often conflicting selves and *towards* being a community within which each and every self can be valued and embraced, celebrating difference where appropriate, rather than demanding absolute conformity and balance – several selves *being as one* rather than *being one self*, if you will.

Carl Rogers wrote of one client, *Mrs Oak*, who described her own process as:

> No longer thinking about my problems or working on them – but enjoying the feeling *process* - and certainly learning something.
> (Rogers 1961: p. 78)

Carl described how, at first, client experiences may be examined by the client without him or her particularly associating them with the self, while later in the counselling process they become assimilated into the client's self structure. Mrs Oak described her therapy as a kind of 'song without words', a kind of poem, only to become dismissive of this, discounting or 'writing off' her experience as an unacceptable form of self-indulgence. All too often the therapist hears clients say things like there being so many other people 'out there' far more deserving of help than the client him- or herself, other people with far more serious problems, concerns and situations. Very often clients report that they feel 'bad' about 'wasting the therapist's time' and feel guilt and shame about this focus on their selves. Yet such feelings and thoughts meet with authentic therapist respect (which does not mean that the therapist agrees with the client) and empathic understanding (not reassurance), and as a consequence clients tend to move into a new phase – one that Rogers summarised as follows:

> *I came here to solve problems, and now I find myself just experiencing myself.*
> (Rogers 1961: p. 80)

Mrs Oak said that it was somewhat akin to blind people learning Braille – that is, it was like *learning a new way of experiencing*. There follows a shift *away from* mechanical or *practical problem solving* and *doing* and *towards being* a *process* of *experiencing*. At a cognitive or intellectual level, clients often report that the experiencing of experiencing somehow seems 'wrong' (hence the feelings of guilt or shame), and yet *at an experiential level the experiencing of experiencing feels good*. It may well be that early in the therapeutic process this experiencing of experience is a kind of free-flowing, 'go for it', 'no holds barred – just be it' way of being, because it feels so good, so new, so unusual, so different, and so liberating that clients really revel in it. However, as therapy progresses, more attention is paid by the client to exploring and organising this experiencing, and then assimilating or incorporating their self-discoveries into the self-concept.

The full experiencing of an affectional relationship

A second characteristic of client-centred therapeutic process is:

> the learning, on the part of the client, to accept fully and freely and without fear *the positive feelings of another*.
> (Rogers 1961: pp. 80–1)

Research findings indicated that this learning does not occur in every single client-centred therapeutic experience, although it is more frequent in long-term counselling – yet even then the pattern is not uniform. However, this learning *is* more likely to be a feature of *successful* therapy. The full experiencing of an affectional relationship is *deep* and *significant*, and yet it is often *not verbalised*. For Mrs Oak, for instance:

> This letting the counsellor and his warm interest into her life was *undoubtedly one of the deepest features of therapy*.
> (Rogers 1961: p. 81)

Carl Rogers wrote that the phenomenon of clients fully receiving therapist unconditional positive regard is definitely *not* one of transference and counter-transference. Rather, it is something *mutual* and *appropriate* (whereas so-called transference and counter-transference are characteristically one-way and inappropriate to the 'realities' of the situation). Rogers believed that there was a discernible trend towards client-centred therapists becoming less afraid of their positive (and negative) feelings towards clients (which in turn may be linked with more activities aimed at increasing therapist *congruence*). For example, at the beginning of therapy the client-centred counsellor *receives* clients with a deep respect for their innate *potential*:

> As a result [the therapist] feels toward the client a warm, positive, affectional reaction. This poses a problem for the client who often . . . finds it difficult to accept the positive feeling of another. Yet once accepted the inevitable reaction on the part of the client is to relax, to let the warmth of liking by another person reduce the tension and fear involved in facing life.
>
> (Rogers 1961: p. 82)

As tension and fear dissipate, so the therapeutic process unfolds, and the attitude of the therapist becomes more one of *awe* as the counsellor is witness to a process that is experienced like watching a beautiful butterfly emerging from a chrysalis, or seeing a foal determinedly taking its first few stumbling steps, or a newly hatched baby turtle struggling to reach the sea. Indeed, Carl Rogers wrote that being with the awesome actualising of potential can engender far deeper feelings of connection – not just with or to the client but with the whole brotherhood and sisterhood of human beings, or even a kind of universal, spiritual connection and sense of belonging.

Yet being in awe of clients is, according to Carl Rogers, not quite the same as feeling *love*, for he stated that profound unconditional positive regard is even more basic or fundamental than love, sexual desires or parental commitments to children.

> It is the simple outgoing human feeling of one individual for another . . . caring enough about the person that you do not wish to interfere with [another's] development, nor to use [others] for any self-aggrandizing goals of your own. Your satisfaction comes in having set others free to grow in [their] own fashion.
>
> (Rogers 1961: p. 84)

We have seen that on entering therapy clients are likely to be vulnerable, anxious, incongruent, defensive, and lacking in self-esteem. Thus clients are likely to believe that they do not deserve or merit being respected or prized by others. They especially do not believe that they merit *unconditional* prizing. Most if not all of their relationships up until now will have been *conditional*, not unconditional, so this experiencing with their therapist may well be something clients feel that they have never received, or at least a quality they have no recollection of ever having experienced. Clients may also try to minimise the significance of their therapist to them, for prizing from a significant other is threatening. If a client's self-concept (largely constructed around introjected conditions of worth) dictates to them that they are not worthy of being openly and freely valued, then there will understandably follow a defence against the full receiving of therapist unconditional positive regard. However:

> To discover that it is *not* devastating to accept the positive feeling from another, that it does not necessarily end in hurt, that it actually 'feels good' to have another person with you in your struggles to meet life – this may be one of the most profound learnings encountered by the individual, whether in therapy or not.
>
> (Rogers 1961: p. 85)

This aspect of the process does not end here – for if a client becomes openly able to experience therapist unconditional positive regard (that is, if there is no longer a defensive need to protect the self-concept by denying or distorting perceptions of being unconditionally valued) then, as a consequence, the client becomes more able to value others. Rogers summarised this by writing that:

> It appears possible that one of the characteristics of deep or significant therapy is that the client discovers that it is not devastating to admit fully into his own experience the positive feeling which another, the therapist, holds towards him. Perhaps one of the reasons why this is so difficult is that essentially it involves the feeling that 'I am worthy of being liked' . . . This aspect of therapy is a free and full experiencing of an affectional relationship which may be put in generalized terms as follows: 'I can permit someone to care about me, and can fully accept that caring within myself. This permits me to recognise that I care, and care deeply, for and about others'.
>
> (Rogers 1961: p. 86)

Thus in early process stages the client might distort the experiencing of unconditional positive regard from their therapist by being cynical (for instance, their therapist is being paid to like them, or is simply being professional and doing his or her job). To admit that I am a person worthy of the effort of a significant other trying to respectfully understand me might be very threatening to the concept of self. Yet once I can *allow* myself to be unconditionally prized, I discover that I, too, can allow myself to care deeply and unconditionally about others.

The liking of one's self

So in successful client-centred therapy, *negative self-attitudes decrease* and *positive self-attitudes increase* – there is a gradual *increase in self-acceptance* and a correlated *increase in acceptance of others*. However, Rogers wrote that such statements do not entirely or accurately portray the complete picture, as they could be interpreted as implying a *grudging* or *reluctant* acceptance, whereas in successful client-centred therapy the client not only becomes more accepting of self, but actually comes to *like* that self. Carl qualified this statement, too, when he wrote that:

> This is not a bragging or self-assertive liking; it is rather a quiet pleasure in *being* one's self.
>
> (Rogers 1961: p. 87)

This process *may* be a consequence of the full experiencing of an affectional relationship, the experiencing in full awareness of therapist unconditional positive regard and empathic understanding. There may be a sense of spontaneity or of relaxation, of enjoyment or a 'primitive joie de vivre' – a basic appreciation of *being oneself*. It is possible that this is a way of being that clients *rediscover* rather than something new that is discovered (that is, if self-actualising has served to thwart the actualising tendency, reconnecting with the actualising tendency may well feel like a 'new' experience). Carl Rogers made references to analogies such as the frisky, gamboling lamb, and the playful dolphin leaping and splashing in the water, in an attempt to capture this joyful awakening.

Very often when clients enter therapy they soon disclose that they feel 'dysfunctional' or that they 'don't even know who the real me is' any more, or that they are 'in pieces' and broken – a kind of 'I'm not working properly any more' theme. However, this can move towards experiencing themselves as more healthy, whole, 'functional' people who, rather than rejecting, denying, suppressing or distorting their feelings can actually *be* and *live* them. Carl Rogers stated that this is:

> an important and often overlooked truth about the therapeutic process. It works in the direction of permitting the person to experience fully, and in awareness, all of his reactions including his feelings and emotions. As this occurs, the individual feels a positive liking for himself, a genuine appreciation of himself as a total functioning unit, which is one of the important *end points* of therapy.
>
> (Rogers 1961: p. 90)

The discovery that the core of personality is positive

Carl Rogers wrote that:

> One of the most revolutionary concepts to grow out of our clinical experience is the growing recognition that the innermost core of man's nature, the deepest layers of his personality, the base of his 'animal nature', is positive in nature – is basically *socialised, forward-moving, rational* and *realistic*.
>
> (Rogers 1961: pp. 90–1)

Rogers did not expect his findings to be accepted by our modern culture. Most major religions, for instance, permeate societies with the concept that we are all fundamentally sinful and in need of either punishment, forgiveness or repentance – and that only by something akin to a miracle (or death) can we become inherently good. We have to be saved from our inner natures. Likewise in the so-called 'caring' professions, where the influence of Sigmund Freud and his psychoanalytic followers, for example, indicated that if the 'id' enshrined within us were to be uncontrolled or unrestrained, the resultant mayhem would be catastrophic. Behaviourists, too, seemed to see people as things to be restrained, controlled and managed, and more cognitive approaches set about correcting our faulty thinking. Overwhelmingly, whether it be religion or psychology, *people simply could not be trusted to direct their own lives.* Carl Rogers therefore instigated thorough research activities in an attempt to validate his deeply held views based on his own experiences as a client-centred psychotherapist. Of religions and psychoanalysis he wrote:

> The whole problem of therapy, as seen by this group, is how to hold these untamed forces in check in a wholesome and constructive manner, rather than in the costly fashion of the neurotic.
>
> (Rogers 1961: p. 91)

Furthermore, such views that at heart human beings are irrational, unsocialised, self-destructive and destructive of others tended to be (and perhaps still are, by many) accepted without question. Although his own beliefs could be seen as radical and revolutionary, blasphemous or just plain wrong, Rogers was not entirely alone. He was able to quote Abraham Maslow, for instance, who posited that 'anti-social' emotions (such as hostility and jealousy) result from the *frustration* of *more basic impulses* for love, security and belonging, which are in themselves desirable. Rogers also referred to Montagu, who postulated that *co-operation*, rather than struggle, is the basic law of human life. Yet the alleged 'caring' resources of so-called 'advanced' societies seemed to serve to 'keep us under control' or 'keep us under cover', or both. Rogers stated that *of course* hostile and anti-social feelings are continually uncovered in counselling, yet must one therefore assume that these indicate that our deeper and therefore basic natures are somehow 'bad' or even 'evil'? Rogers believed that feelings associated with hostility (or feelings that are deemed to be 'anti-social') were not representative of either our deepest or even our strongest essence. Rather:

> the inner core of man's personality is the organism itself, which is essentially both *self-preserving* and *social*.
>
> (Rogers 1961: p. 92)

In the case of Mrs Oak, beneath her first layer of defence lay *bitterness* and a *desire* for *revenge*. A 'murderous feeling of hatred and a desire to get even' was behind the 'socially controlled surfaces of her behaviour'. Considerably later on (after 23 sessions), Mrs Oak returned to this theme, this time feeling somewhat emotionally blocked, and when the 'barriers burst', the feeling has become *less* anti-social and more like a 'desire to get back at the world which has cheated her, a deep experience of having been hurt'. At this deeper level, it is very clear indeed that she had no desire to put her murderous feelings into action. In fact, she *disliked* those feelings and *wished to be rid of them*. Three sessions later, 'reaching far down into herself', the following consecutive themes were expressed:

> I'm going to talk about myself as *self*-ish
> but with a new connotation to the word.
>
> I've acquired an acquaintance with the structure of myself,
> *know myself* deeply.
>
> As I descend into myself, I discover something exciting,
> a *core* that is *totally without hate*.
>
> It can't be a part of everyday life – it may even be *abnormal*.
>
> I thought first it was just a *sublimated sex drive*.
>
> But no, this is more *inclusive, deeper* than sex.
>
> One would expect this to be the kind of thing one would discover
> by going up into the thin realms of *ideals*.
>
> It seems to be something that is the *essence* that lasts.
>
> (Rogers 1961: pp. 99–100)

This almost 'mystical' client summary, by the next session, has become clearer, more concise, and the *difficulty of the experiencing is acknowledged* by the client. Rogers wrote:

> Her feeling goes against the grain of her culture, [yet] she feels bound
> to say that the *core* of herself is *not bad, nor terribly wrong*, but something
> *positive. Underneath* the layer of *controlled surface behaviour*, underneath
> the *bitterness*, underneath the *hurt*, [underneath the murderous hate
> and desire for revenge] is a *self that is positive*, and that is *without hate.*
> This I believe is the lesson which our clients have been facing us with
> for a long time, and which we have been slow to learn.
>
> (Rogers 1961: p. 101)

The deeper one digs into oneself, the less one has to fear. Instead of discovering
'bad' or 'terribly wrong', there is a core self which is deeply socialised, without
hate, and wanting to neither punish nor reward others.

In looking at 'negative', 'aggressive' or 'hostile' aspects of human behaviour, at
this point I turn from Carl's narrative about Mrs Oak towards my own experience.
After thousands upon thousands of client hours, I can state that *not once* have I
ever experienced anger, rage, hostility or aggression as being at the core of, or
being the essential essence of, a human being. *Inevitably* there were other factors
underlying and generating such apparently 'negative' emotions and thoughts.
Take anger, for instance. In terms of the belief system that forms a significant part
of a self-concept, there was often the thought that something was unfair or
unjust. Outrage at injustice may not only be an understandable reaction, it might
even be considered honourable (and hence acceptable or even highly desirable)
in certain contexts. Who decides which contexts make anger at injustice acceptable or unacceptable? Let us say, however, that in one particular instance the
perceived injustice seems 'irrational' or 'unreasonable' – maybe exhibited by a
'selfish' individual who is seemingly unable to see past or beyond their own needs
and desires, and to hell with anyone else. Is this person inherently bad? Or might
this person feel deprived of the love and affection that they had been led to
believe was their birthright?

Quite often when engaging in a debate about the basic nature of human
beings, someone will say 'Ah . . . but what about Hitler? How can anyone
conceivably say that he was innately good?'. Well, personally I cannot conceive
that Adolf Hitler was inherently bad at the time he was conceived! I wonder, for
instance, how things might have been if this young Adolf, with his creative flair
and artistic temperament, had not been so cruelly rejected (as he perceived it)
for art college.

Being one's organism, one's experience

The client-centred approach to therapy, Carl Rogers wrote, is:

> a process whereby man *becomes* his organism – *without self-deception,
> without distortion.*
>
> (Rogers 1961: p. 103)

It is because this process and its outcomes are *experiential* (a way of being) that it
does not readily lend itself to accurate symbolisation in words alone. Indeed, Carl
stated that if this experience were to be understood in words alone, this would be
but an abstract from or a distortion of the totality of this way of being (in the way
that a map of a piece of land is not the territory itself). Yet we try. There is a sense in

which the process of client-centred therapy is towards a rediscovery of what once was – getting back in touch with the organismic valuing process that reigned prior to the onset of a concept of self that was formulated through introjected values and the sometimes tyrannical rule of consequent conditions of worth. Historically, *prior to* the advent of client-centred therapy, clients might have asked themselves things like 'What do others think I should do?', 'What would my parents suggest that I should do?', 'What would my culture tell me to do?' and 'What do I think I should or ought to do?'. Yet clients may not necessarily *act* in or *be in accord with* the 'shoulds' and 'oughts' of others (individually or as groups). Even when in rebellion against external loci of evaluation, the person is nevertheless *acting in terms of those external expectations*, and often those expectations have been *introjected into the self-concept*. (I am reminded of the woman who, having felt liberated from a lousy relationship for some months, suddenly froze in the middle of a clothes-shopping expedition. She suddenly realised that she was buying exactly the opposite of what she used to buy for, or on behalf of, her ex-partner. It struck her like a thunderbolt that actually it was the ex-partner's values that were still the governing factor, only this time it was in opposition to them. She was dumbstruck as she realised that she did not know what she herself liked.)

During client-centred therapy, clients are more likely to ask 'How do I *experience* this?' and 'What does it *mean* to me?' and 'If I behave in a certain way, *how do I symbolise the meaning* which it will have for me?'. Rogers termed this openness to experiencing and the accurate perception and symbolisation of that experiencing *'realism'*, in the sense that the person is able to access all significant valuing and achieve a realistic 'balance' based on this absence of denial or distortion. It does seem that a great deal of human energy is expended on trying to be, feel and do in a consistent manner. For instance, the recently bereaved should only feel sorrow, even if a part of them (no matter how small) perhaps feels a sense of relief at being unburdened from an exhausting and inconvenient duty of care. If this feeling of relief is admitted to awareness (that is, if it is symbolised in consciousness), it is accompanied by deep guilt for being so shameful, callous and selfish as to have an emotion that one is not expected to feel. Rogers gave several of his own examples, including the following:

> I have thought I must feel only *love* for my parents, but I find that I experience both love and *bitter resentment*. Perhaps I can be that person who *freely experiences both love and resentment*.

And:

> I have thought I was only *bad* and *worthless*. Now I experience myself at times as one of *much worth* – at other times as one of *little worth* or usefulness. Perhaps I can be a person who *experiences varying degrees of worth*.
>
> (Rogers 1961: p. 104)

For another client:

> I have held the conception that *no-one could really love me for myself*. Now I experience the *affective warmth of another* for me. Perhaps I can be a person who is *loveable by others* – perhaps I *am* such a person.
>
> (Rogers 1961: p. 104)

And for yet another:

> I have been brought up to feel that *I must not appreciate myself – but do.* I
> can *cry* for myself, but I can *enjoy* myself, too. Perhaps *I am a richly
> varied person* whom I can enjoy and for whom I can feel sorry.
>
> (Rogers 1961: p. 104)

Mrs Oak said:

> I have thought that in some deep way I was *bad,* that the most basic
> elements in me must be *dire* and *awful.* I don't *experience* that *badness*
> but rather a *positive desire to live and let live. Perhaps I can be that person
> who is, at heart, positive.*
>
> (Rogers 1961: p. 104)

Rogers believed that a fundamental ingredient that makes much of this process of
becoming possible is complete and free *awareness of experiencing.* There is an
elimination (or at least minimising) of *denial and distortion to awareness.* There is an
awareness of *what is actually experienced* through all of the body and mind ('sensory
and visceral' experiencing) – not simply the crumbs that are left over after our
needs to defend our self-concepts (and conditions of worth) have screened out or
filtered our experience in an attempt to either 'make it fit' or deny it altogether.
This, then, is about *realising full potential,* with:

> the enriching element of awareness freely added to the basic aspect of
> sensory and visceral reaction. The person comes to *be* what he *is,* as
> clients so frequently say in therapy . . . the individual comes to *be* – in
> *awareness* – what he *is* - in experience. He is, in other words, a *complete
> and fully functioning human organism.*
>
> (Rogers 1961: pp. 104–5)

Carl Rogers was very passionate about what he saw as the appalling way in which
people had hitherto been treated in the name of health, based on socialised beliefs
that we are all inherently 'bad' and untrustworthy. He wrote that:

> When a man is *less* than fully man – when he *denies to awareness* various
> aspects of his experience – then indeed we have all too often reason to
> fear him and his behaviour, as the present world situation testifies.
>
> (Rogers 1961: p. 105)

In other words, if we believe that we are by our very innermost natures evil or
hostile or murderous or licentious, then we are likely to treat ourselves and each
other in ways designed to prevent our animalistic ways holding sway. Yet Rogers
believed that:

> There is no beast in man. There is only man in man, and this we have
> been able to release.
>
> (Rogers 1961: p. 105)

If we can dare to believe that our innermost natures, based on a constructive
actualising tendency, are actually *positive* in nature, then rather than control,
manage, manipulate, educate, change or suppress the human psyche, our innate

potential becomes open to being *released* (through the provision of appropriate conditions). Here then is a real message of hope:

> If we can *add to* the sensory and visceral experiencing which is characteristic of the whole animal kingdom, the gift of a *free and undistorted awareness* of which only the human animal seems fully capable, we have an organism which is *beautifully and constructively realistic*. We have then an organism which is as *aware* of the demands of the culture as it is of its own physiological demands for food or sex – which is just as *aware* of its desire for friendly relationships as it is of its desire to aggrandize itself – which is just as *aware* of its delicate and sensitive tenderness toward others, as it is of its hostilities toward others. When man's *unique capacity of awareness* is thus functioning freely and fully, we find that we have not an animal whom we must fear, not a beast who must be controlled, but an organism *able to achieve*, through the remarkable integrative capacity of its central nervous system, a *balanced, realistic, self-enhancing, other-enhancing* behaviour as a resultant of all these elements of *awareness*.
>
> (Rogers 1961: p. 105)

Carl believed that 'fully functioning' people are to be *trusted* and that their behaviour is *constructive*. In today's world, fully functioning people might not be perceived as entirely conventional and they might not always blindly conform to accepted norms and mores, yet Rogers believed that by our very natures we are both individuals (and hence individualised) and social beings (and hence socialised). He also acknowledged the difference between *deep conviction* and *truth*. He wrote of his own deep truths, and asked readers to look deep inside themselves and see whether or not the deep convictions of Carl Rogers resonate within.

Therapist be

If the therapist initiates certain conducive conditions, *then* a process can unfold in which the innate potential of human beings may be released. Carl Rogers stated that:

> In client-centered therapy we are deeply engaged in the prediction and influencing of behavior, or even the control of behavior. As therapists, we institute certain attitudinal conditions, and the client has relatively little voice in the establishment of these conditions. We predict that if these conditions are instituted, certain behavioral consequences will ensue in the client.
>
> (Rogers and Evans 1975, p. lxxvi)

It is *the therapist* who takes the core conditions to the relationship, and *the therapist* who establishes a contact based on those conditions. So, having placed the therapist conditions back together again in Chapter 4, now let us to some degree take them apart again! As we move through these conditions, they do in fact interface very much throughout.

Congruence and process

The greater the degree of counsellor congruence (that is, congruence between experience, awareness, and communication), the more likely it is that the client will experience *clear* and therapeutic communication. If all verbal, paraverbal and non-verbal therapist expressions spring from congruence and unity, then there is much less likelihood that these cues will have an ambiguous or unclear meaning to the client. In order to achieve relatively high degrees of congruence, therapists need to listen to themselves, to get in touch with their own inner, complex, diverse and ever-changing attitudes and feelings, and to hear themselves with *acceptance* – as Rogers said, to become more adequate at *being* the person you *are*, and that just as clients need to feel received in order to grow, so therapist self-acceptance is necessary for personal growth.

The more clearly the counsellor communicates, the more *the client* responds to the counsellor with clarity. Thus even though clients are likely to be relatively incongruent, nevertheless their responses will have *more* clarity and congruence than would be the case if the counsellor's communications were themselves incongruent, confusing or ambiguous. The greater the degree of counsellor congruence (for instance, the less the counsellor is presenting a professional façade or a role that has to be defended), the less need there is for that counsellor to be defensive, and hence the greater the counsellor's ability to listen accurately and hear the client. This links *congruence* to *empathic understanding*, because at least to this degree clients feel empathically understood – that whether client expressions have been defensive or congruent, the counsellor has understood clients more or less as they see themselves. This also links congruence and empathic understanding to *unconditional positive regard*, as the client who feels really heard and to some degree understood (which is a consequence of the counsellor respecting the client) is likely to experience positive feelings (regard) *towards their counsellor* (the mutual respect and understanding that Rogers called 'the experiencing of an affectional relationship'). As a consequence of this there are fewer barriers to communication – the need for defensiveness gradually decreases. In other words, it is therapeutic if clients experience their therapists as real:

> I would like my feelings in this relationship with him to be as clear and transparent as possible, so that they are a discernible reality for him, to which he can return again and again . . . I recognize that this is a very human and unpredictable journey for me, as well as for him, and that I may, without even knowing my fear, shrink away within myself, from some of the feelings he discovers. To this extent I know I will be limited in my ability to help him. I realize that at times his own fears may make him perceive me as uncaring, as rejecting, as an intruder, as one who does not understand. I want fully to accept these feelings in him, and yet I hope also that my own real feelings will show through so clearly that in time he cannot fail to perceive them. Most of all I want him to encounter in me a real person. I do not need to be uneasy as to whether my own feelings are 'therapeutic'. What I am and what I feel are good enough to be a basis for therapy, if I can transparently *be* what I am and what I feel in relationship to him. Then perhaps he can be what he is, openly and without fear.

And the client, for his part, goes through far more complex sequences which can only be suggested. Perhaps schematically his feelings change in some of these ways. 'I'm afraid of him. I want help, but I don't know whether to trust him. He might see things which I don't know in myself – frightening and bad elements. He seems not to be judging me, but I'm sure he is. I can't tell him what really concerns me, but I can tell him about some past experiences which are related to my concern. He seems to understand those, so I can reveal a bit more of myself. But now that I've shared with him some of this bad side of me, he despises me. I'm sure of it, but it's strange I can find little evidence of it. Do you suppose that what I've told him isn't so bad? Is it possible that I need not be ashamed of it as a part of me? I no longer feel that he despises me. It makes me feel that I want to go further, exploring *me*, perhaps expressing more of myself. I find him a sort of companion as I do this – he seems really to understand.

But now I'm getting frightened again, and this time deeply frightened. I didn't realize that exploring the unknown recesses of myself would make me feel feelings I've never experienced before. It's very strange because in one way these aren't new feelings. I sense that they've always been there. But they seem so bad and disturbing I've never dared to let them flow in me. And now as I live these feelings in the hours with him, I feel terribly shaky, as though my world is falling apart. It used to be sure and firm. Now it is loose, permeable and vulnerable. It isn't pleasant to feel things I've always been frightened of before. It's his fault. Yet curiously I'm eager to see him and I feel more safe when I'm with him.

I don't know who I am any more, but sometimes when I *feel* things I seem solid and real for a moment. I'm troubled by the contradictions I find in myself – I act one way and feel another – I think one thing and feel another. It's very disconcerting. It's also sometimes adventurous and exhilarating to be trying to discover who I am. Sometimes I catch myself feeling that perhaps the person I am is worth being, whatever that means.

I'm beginning to find it very satisfying, though often painful, to share just what it is I'm feeling at this moment. You know, it is really helpful to try to listen to myself, to hear what is going on in me. I'm not so frightened any more of what *is* going on in me. It seems pretty trustworthy. I use some of my hours with him to dig deep into myself to know what I *am* feeling. It's scary work, but I want to *know*. And I do trust him most of the time, and that helps. I feel pretty vulnerable and raw, but I know he doesn't want to hurt me, and I even believe he cares. It occurs to me as I try to let myself down and down, deep into myself, that maybe if I could sense what is going on in me, and could realize its meaning, I would know who I am, and I would also know what to do. At least I feel this knowing sometimes with him.

I can even tell him just how I'm feeling toward him at any given moment and instead of this killing the relationship, as I used to fear, it seems to deepen it. Do you suppose I could be my feelings with other people also? Perhaps that wouldn't be too dangerous either.

You know, I feel as if I'm floating along on the current of life, very adventurously, being me. I get defeated sometimes, I get hurt sometimes, but I'm learning that those experiences are not fatal. I don't *know* exactly *who* I am, but I can feel my reactions at any given moment, and they seem to work out pretty well as a basis for my behavior from moment to moment. Maybe this is what it *means* to be *me*. But of course I can only do this because I feel safe in the relationship with my therapist. Or could I be myself this way outside of this relationship? I wonder. I wonder. Perhaps I could . . .'.

(Rogers 1961: pp. 67–9)

Thus clients are now able to hear themselves *and* receive the communications from their counsellor more clearly, and hence the process of reciprocal empathy has been established.

This means that to some degree the process of therapy occurs in each and that the outcomes of therapy will to that same degree occur in each; change in personality in the direction of greater unity and integration; less conflict and more energy utilizable for effective living; change in behaviour in the direction of greater maturity.

(Rogers 1961: p. 344)

Relating congruence to interpersonal communication, Carl Rogers proposed a 'tentative statement of a general law' stating that, assuming an ongoing minimal willingness to be in contact and receive communication from each other:

The greater the congruence of experience, awareness and communication on the part of one individual, the more the ensuing relationship will involve: a tendency toward reciprocal communication with a quality of increasing congruence; a tendency toward more mutually accurate understanding of the communications; improved psychological adjustment and functioning in both parties; mutual satisfaction in the relationship.

(Rogers 1961: p. 344)

It follows that the opposite is true, too – that the greater the *incongruence* of the therapist, the greater the 'disintegration' of accurate empathic understanding, resulting in psychological 'maladjustment' and hence a dissatisfying therapeutic relationship for both counsellor and client.

Congruence: Fay, an illustration

Fay was referred for counselling by her GP, having 'fallen apart' as a consequence of the termination of a relationship. She was in torment, with one part (her self-structure) trying its best to convince another part (a part that was desperately yearning to be with her partner again) that actually she was better off without him – battle was raging within.

Let me be honest here: I abhor violence and aggression in whatever way, shape or form – I am a confirmed pacifist and coward, and proud of being both. Therefore one judgement would be that *of course* Fay would be better off without her former partner, for he sounded like a 'nasty piece of work'! However, to voice such an opinion within the therapy session would not have been congruent, as my client-centred *discipline* means that while such an opinion might very fleetingly enter my mind (mostly due to a physiological reaction of disgust at some of his reported behaviour), my primary commitment is to strive to enter *Fay's* world of feelings and meanings. My anti-violence values are neither denied nor distorted in the moment – they are simply irrelevant, or at least relatively irrelevant in relation to Fay's world of feelings and meanings. Perhaps the notion of taking precedence might illustrate client-centred discipline. In counselling, the client's frame of reference *takes precedence over* the counsellor's frame of reference. If there is no psychological denial or distortion on the part of the therapist, unconditional positive regard, in large part communicated through empathic understanding, remains authentic and is largely communicated through being empathic.

Unconditional positive regard and process

To begin with, Carl Rogers wrote that.

> When the therapist is experiencing a positive, acceptant attitude toward whatever the client is at that moment, therapeutic movement or change is more likely to occur.
>
> (Rogers 1980: p. 116)

This view that the client experiencing respect from the counsellor was therapeutically helpful moved from being a *belief* in the early days into being a therapeutic value based on solid experience and data, for:

> Research indicates that the more this attitude is experienced by the therapist, the greater the probability that therapy will be successful.
>
> (Rogers 1978: p. 10)

So what is this change that is more likely to occur if clients experience unconditional positive regard, and how might this change occur?

> In therapy, with its climate of acceptance and safety and its freedom to explore one's feelings whatever they may be, it becomes possible for the client to experience the feelings that have not been admitted into his concept of self. Once experienced in an accepting climate, they can gradually be incorporated into his self-picture, and he thereby achieves more unity and integration between the person he organismically is and the self he perceives himself as being.
>
> (Rogers 1989: p. 24)

Thus we can see that client experiencing of unconditional positive regard from the therapist enables the client to inwardly go where they may not have been before. There is a hitherto unexperienced freedom to explore the self:

> When the counselor perceives and accepts the client as he is, when he lays aside all evaluation and enters into the perceptual frame of reference of the client, he frees the client to explore his life and

experience anew, frees him to perceive in that experience new meanings and new goals.

(Rogers 1951: p. 48)

As a consequence of this freedom to self-explore in an acceptant climate, self-perceptions may change and be incorporated into a new and ever-changing 'picture' of the self. However, Rogers said:

> I believe that the person can only accept the unacceptable in himself when he is in a close relationship in which he experiences acceptance. This, I think, is a large share of what constitutes psychotherapy – that the individual finds that the feelings he has been ashamed of or that he has been unable to admit into his awareness, that those can be accepted by another person, so then he becomes able to accept them as a part of himself.

> (Rogers 1951: p. 71)

As we have seen, the client-centred therapist does not have to be *perfect* in this experiencing of respect that clients perceive – if this were so, there would be no client-centred therapists. Yet we have also already encountered the conviction that *imperfect* human beings can be of help (especially if they are aware and accepting of their imperfections). Although it may be true that more empathy is better than some, and some is better than none, at the heart of the empathic process is a therapist who is *striving* to understand:

> The accuracy of the therapist's empathic understanding has often been emphasised, but more important is the therapist's *interest* in appreciating the world of the client and offering such understanding with the willingness to be corrected. This creates a process in which the therapist gets closer and closer to the client's meanings and feelings, developing an ever-deepening relationship based on respect for and understanding of the other person.
> (Rogers and Raskin 1989: p. 171)

Thus the therapist attitude of unconditional positive regard precedes empathic understanding in the necessary and sufficient conditions because any understanding is born out of the genuine desire to understand, based on a belief that people are worth the effort. This desire and genuine interest, as we have seen in Chapter 4, is ongoing through each moment.

> Acceptance does not mean much until it involves understanding. It is only as I *understand* the feelings and thoughts which seem so horrible to you, or so weak, or so sentimental, or so bizarre – it is only as I see them as you see them, and accept them and you, that you feel really free to explore all the hidden nooks and frightening crannies of your inner and often buried experience. This *freedom* is an important condition of the relationship. There is implied here a freedom to explore oneself at both conscious and unconscious levels, as rapidly as one can dare to embark on this dangerous quest.
> (Rogers 1961: p. 34)

Here, then, we see an interweave between respect and empathy. Respect is communicated through a belief that the other person is worth the effort of striving to understand, and without understanding that respect means little. The therapist appreciates the client enough to want to understand, and, as the client reveals more, and as each disclosure meets with non-evaluative unconditional positive regard and a degree of empathic understanding, further respect is evident as the therapist strives to respectfully engage with and understand this untangling client.

While it has been stressed that the client-centred therapist does not intend to offer support, clients may well nevertheless experience the counselling relationship as supportive, because they will feel *prized* through perceiving the therapist's attitude of unconditional positive regard and consequent striving to empathise – an attitude that is based at least in part upon a belief in the primacy of the actualising tendency, and the right and capacity of clients to self-direction and dignity. Thus one consequence of sensitive and respectful empathy is that it helps to *dissolve feelings of alienation*, because the client feels deeply accepted as the person he or she is from moment to moment:

> A second consequence of empathic understanding is that the recipient feels valued, cared for, accepted as the person that he or she is . . . It is impossible to accurately sense the perceptual world of another person unless you value that person and his or her world – unless you, in some sense, care. Hence, the message comes through to the recipient that 'this other individual trusts me, thinks I'm worthwhile. Perhaps I *am* worth something. Perhaps *I* could value *myself.* Perhaps I could care for myself'. It is, I believe, the therapist's caring understanding . . . which has permitted this client to experience a high regard, even a love, for himself.
>
> (Rogers 1980: p. 152)

Remember that Carl Rogers believed that it was *impossible* for a judgemental therapist to perceive a client's world of feelings and meanings with accuracy.

Thus we begin to see some of the process consequences of respectful empathic understanding. Through the client perceiving the attitude of unconditional positive regard that underpins the therapist's striving to understand, there is a tendency for feelings of alienation to dissolve, an increase in client positive self-regard, and an increase in client self-acceptance.

The following quote demonstrates why Carl Rogers believed unconditional positive regard to be a necessary precursor to empathic understanding:

> In the emotional warmth of the relationship with the therapist, the client begins to experience a feeling of safety as he finds that whatever attitude he expresses is understood in almost the same way that he perceives it, and is accepted. He then is able to explore, for example, a vague feeling of guiltiness which he has experienced. In this safe relationship he can perceive for the first time the hostile meaning and purpose of certain aspects of his behavior, and can understand why he has felt guilty about it, and why it has been necessary to deny to awareness the meaning of this behavior. But this clearer perception is in itself disrupting and anxiety-creating, not therapeutic. It is evidence

to the client that there are disturbing inconsistencies in himself, that he is not what he thinks he is. But as he voices his new perceptions and their attendant anxieties, he finds that this acceptant alter ego, the therapist, this other person who is only partly another person, perceives these experiences too, but with a new quality. The therapist perceives the client's self as the client has known it, and accepts it; he perceives the contradictory aspects which have been denied to aware-ness and accepts those too as being a part of the client; and both of these acceptances have in them the same warmth and respect. Thus it is that the client, experiencing in another an acceptance of both these aspects of himself, can take toward himself the same attitude. He finds that he too can accept himself even with the additions and alterations that are necessitated by these new perceptions of himself as hostile. He can experience himself as a person having hostile as well as other types of feelings, and can experience himself in this way without guilt. He has been enabled to do this (if our theory is correct) because another person has been able to adopt his frame of reference, to perceive with him, yet to perceive with acceptance and respect.

(Rogers 1951: p. 41)

Unconditional positive regard: Fay, an illustration

It felt very important that Fay's yearning to be with her ex-partner be heard, accepted and understood if she were to feel fully received and therefore free to move on, so the therapist conditions easily took precedence over any extraneous thoughts or opinions that, albeit momentarily, I may have had. Fay was not at all accepting of the desperately yearning part of herself. Indeed, every time she made reference to this aspect of herself, words like 'silly, stupid, crazy and mad' were mentioned – and she herself felt that this part of her needed to be defeated, crushed, exiled or even killed. Yet if I had also judged this part of her to be unworthy (or if I had somehow colluded with or condoned her value judgements about herself), then in effect her *whole person* would not have been welcomed into therapy.

Metaphorically speaking, a barrier burst during the ninth session, and Fay felt able to use the entire 50 minutes to disclose how she had engaged in 'perverse, often brutal, sexual activities' with her ex-partner. Although as part of her 'ex-orcism' Fay needed to be sexually explicit, I shall not be. Suffice it to say that physically she would lose handfuls of hair and end up severely battered and bruised as a consequence of these episodes. Worse still for her, very often she would 'willingly' go along with or even instigate these hideous sex sessions. Fay felt shame and embarrassment, and she felt violated and defiled – yet how could she be angry or blame her ex-partner when she had *apparently* so willingly engaged in this way?

It is my deeply held conviction that had Fay not felt fully received during previous sessions – that is, had her *longing-to-be-with-him-again* self as well as her *better-off-without-him* self not met with compassion, acceptance, respect and understanding, she would not have felt safe and secure enough as a whole person to make the disclosures she did (to a male counsellor, at that).

Both at the time and in retrospect, it was clear that this ninth session was a real turning point for Fay, a truly cathartic experience. She later described how hard it had been for her to disclose such shameful acts and her feeling of being so dirty and unclean, especially as she had co-operated so seemingly fully with her own defilement. Again it felt really important to hear, accept and understand her *I-blame-myself* self, as unless she felt fully received once again she would have been less likely to move on. (I stress that my intent is never to move anyone on – my intent is to strive to be the therapist conditions, and I know that, if I am successful, clients are likely to move on as a consequence.)

In the tenth session, Fay was realising the degree to which she had been manipulated, coerced and exploited by her ex-partner (she had clearly spent a great deal of time in between these two sessions processing her feelings and thoughts). From the moment she arrived (she seemed to breeze into the room rather than trudge) Fay seemed lighter in mood – genuinely smiling at times, for instance, and making more open eye contact – and derogatory riders about her own 'silliness' had all but disappeared. She had remembered how her ex-partner had a video of sexual performances with a previous partner (a 'benchmark' that she was expected to live up to), and she recalled how he would express feeling let down, and would mope or become withdrawn if Fay was not prepared to engage in certain sexual activities (as previous partners had), so that she felt as if she really was the huge disappointment her partner made her out to be. Fay was able to recall many, many examples of the 'emotional blackmail' that had been used on her. This time though she approached her self (or selves) with compassionate understanding rather than self-blame, also being able to locate her way of being in time (that is, she was developing a kind of extensional congruence).

We can now turn to empathic understanding and process.

Empathic understanding and process

> The fourth condition for therapy is that the therapist is experiencing an accurate, empathic understanding of the client's world as seen from the inside. To sense the client's private world as if it were your own, but without ever losing the 'as if' quality – this is empathy, and this seems essential to therapy. To sense the client's anger, fear, or confusion as if it were your own, yet without your own anger, fear, or confusion getting bound up in it, is the condition we are endeavoring to describe. When the client's world is this clear to the therapist, and he moves about in it freely, then he can both communicate his understanding of what is clearly known to the client and can also voice meanings in the client's experience of which the client is scarcely aware.
>
> (Rogers 1961: p. 284)

It's just you, you, you all the time!

In a sense, clients are 'all over the place' at the beginning of therapy, while the client-centred counsellor is primarily intent on entering clients' worlds as they see them – hence *you, you, you* . . . However:

> The therapist is not interested in everything equally. He is interested in that which is real, important, significant, or fundamental.
>
> (Barton 1974: p. 191)

And what is most real, important, significant and fundamental to client-centred therapists is the internal frame of reference of clients. How, then, does the process of *beginning* to enter the frame of reference of clients commence? A fundamental striving to hear, understand and voice something of that empathy is a good start, for the experience of Carl Rogers indicated that:

> simply to listen understandingly to a client and to attempt to convey that understanding were potent forces for individual therapeutic change.
>
> (Rogers and Evans 1975: p. 124)

However, the therapist might well face some difficulties in striving to be this way, just one being that:

> much of the client's expression is confused and expressed in such private symbolism that it is difficult to enter into his perceptual field and see experience in his terms.
>
> (Rogers 1951: p. 44)

Rogers pointed out that entering the internal frame of reference of clients is not the 'royal road to learning', and that there are *many* hindrances, another being that the therapist can *mostly* only perceive what is in the conscious awareness of clients, so it follows that the greater the degree of client incongruence, the more incomplete the picture that is available to awareness. Nevertheless:

> If some of that [understanding] can be communicated to the client, that I do really see how you feel and understand the way you feel, that can be a most releasing kind of experience. To find that here is a real person who really accepts and understands sensitively, and accurately perceives just the way the world seems to me – that just seems to pull people forward. The effect that can have is really fascinating. It is this aspect that enables the process of therapy to go on.
>
> (Rogers and Evans 1975: pp. 29–30)

Although Carl wrote of 'empathic inference' and 'empathic guessing', he also cautioned us that:

> The more we try to infer what is present in the phenomenal field but not conscious (as in interpreting projective techniques), the more complex grow the inferences until the interpretation of the client's projections may become merely an illustration of the clinician's projections.
>
> (Rogers 1951: p. 495)

The imperfection of communication is another drawback. We know from our own experience that communicating (verbally, paraverbally and non-verbally) precisely what we think, what we feel, and our personal meanings, is nigh-on impossible – yet in striving to empathically understand clients, client-centred therapists have no choice but to rely on their accurate perceiving of client (verbal, non-verbal and paraverbal) communications. However, the situation is not hopeless. For instance, we can, albeit with some caution, let our own frames of reference be a tentative guide to the world of feelings and meanings of others, for as Rogers wrote:

> It is possible to achieve, to some extent, the other person's frame of reference, because many of the perceptual objects – self, parents, teachers, employers, and so on – have counterparts in our own perceptual field, and practically all the attitudes toward these perceptual objects – such as fear, anger, annoyance, love, jealousy, satisfaction – have been present in our own world of experience . . . Hence we can infer, quite directly, from the communication of the individual, or less accurately from observation of his behaviour, a portion of his perceptual and experiential field.
>
> (Rogers 1951: pp. 495–6)

In process terms, we have seen that the more therapist unconditional positive regard is perceived by clients, the less defensive clients feel that they need to be. The less defensive they feel they need to be, the more experiences become available to conscious awareness and the more free the expression of feelings and meanings becomes. A similar process emerges when therapists offer their empathic perceptions to clients:

> Empathic understanding, when it is accurately and sensitively communicated, seems crucially important in enabling the client more freely to experience his inward feelings, perceptions, and personal meanings. When he is thus in contact with his inward experiencing, he can recognize the points at which his experience is at variance with his concept of himself and, consequently, where he is endeavoring to live by a false conception. Such recognition of incongruence is the first step towards its resolution and the revision of the concept of self to include the hitherto denied experiences. This is one of the major ways in which change becomes possible and a more complete integration of self and behavior is inaugurated.
>
> (Rogers 1989: p. 16)

Given that clients (and especially self-referred clients) are usually motivated towards change in the first place (that is why they sought counselling), it makes a great deal of sense for the therapist to behave in ways that are conducive to clients feeling as free as possible to express and explore themselves:

> It should also be added that the dynamic results – for the client and for the learning of the therapist – which are achieved in client-centred therapy when even a portion of the perceptual field is communicated have led us to feel that here is a way of viewing experience which is much closer to the basic laws of personality process and behaviour. Not only does there result a more vivid understanding of the meaning of behaviour, but the opportunities for new learning are maximized when we approach the individual without a preconceived set of categories which we expect him to fit.
>
> (Rogers 1951: pp. 496–7)

In the process of therapy, a therapist striving to empathise with and understand clients clearly has consequences, one of which is:

> By pointing to the possible meanings in the flow of another person's experiencing, you help the other to focus on this useful type of referent, to experience the meanings more fully, and to move forward in the experiencing.
>
> (Rogers 1980: p. 142)

We have also seen how Carl Rogers believed that empathy, at its best, is mutual in the counselling relationship. Furthemore, he linked this to growth when he said:

> perhaps in the moment where real change takes place, then I wonder if it isn't reciprocal in the sense that I am able to see this individual as he is in that moment and he really sees my understanding and acceptance of him. And that I think is what is reciprocal and is perhaps what produces change.
>
> (Rogers 1989: p. 55)

Carl believed that:

> The whole task of psychotherapy is the task of dealing with a failure in communication.
>
> (Rogers 1961: p. 330)

Thus the process is that incongruent clients have lost their *inner* communication abilities, and this in turn hinders their self-expression (that is, the quality of their relationships with others). Incongruent clients are, due to their defensive psychological denial and distortion mechanisms, no longer consciously aware of certain aspects of their experiencing, and such denial and distortion will of course be reflected in their outer as well as their inner communications. Thus:

> The task of psychotherapy is to help the person achieve, through a special relationship with a therapist, good communication within himself. Once this is achieved he can communicate more freely and more effectively with others. We may say then that psychotherapy is good communication, within and between men. We may also turn that statement around and it will still be true. Good communication, free communication, within or between men, is always therapeutic.
>
> (Rogers 1961: p. 330)

In 1961, when considering group tensions, Carl wrote about how empathic understanding can overcome:

> the insincerities, the defensive exaggerations, the lies, the 'false fronts' which characterize almost every failure in communication.
>
> (Rogers 1961: p. 336)

When people both realise and accept that the sole – the only – authentic intent of the therapist is to respectfully understand, then the need for defensive processes rapidly dissipates. As barriers to both inner and outer communicating dissolve, so clients are enabled to reach their inner truths and engage in more fulsome relationships with others. Rogers likened this movement toward inner truth with accessing data – that is, the more accurate the information one has, the more one is able to make informed, self-directed, responsible choices. For sure, our anxieties, doubts and fears might serve to trigger our defensive processes that are designed to deny us access to the 'facts' yet nevertheless Carl Rogers believed that *the facts in themselves are always friendly*:

> *The facts are friendly* . . . as I look back, it seems to me that I regarded the facts as potential enemies, as possible bearers of disaster. I have perhaps been slow in coming to realize that the facts are *always* friendly. Every bit of evidence one can acquire, in any area, leads one that much closer to what is true. And being closer to the truth can never be a harmful or dangerous or unsatisfying thing. So while I still hate to readjust my thinking, still hate to give up old ways of perceiving and conceptualizing, yet at some deeper level I have, to a considerable degree, come to realize that these painful reorganizations are what is known as *learning*, and that though painful they always lead to a more satisfying because somewhat more accurate way of seeing life.
>
> (Rogers 1961: p. 25)

Having stated that client perception of a therapist's genuine and acceptant empathy helps serve to reduce blocks to communication, it follows that the opposite is true:

> When we don't feel understood, we're defensive.
>
> (Rogers and Teich 1992: p. 59)

An example of this might arise through therapeutic work with couples. All too often, neither partner really hears the other because each is indignantly defending their own stance, and as a consequence neither feels heard or understood. Very often, in the first few sessions with a couple, each client only experiences respectful empathy from the therapist. Very often, couples have later reported how, when they departed from sessions at the beginning of therapy, their conversation was typified by 'See, the counsellor agreed with *me*', 'Oh no! The counsellor was clearly on *my* side!', and so on. In fact the therapist did not *agree* with anyone, but clients reacted in this way to having felt a contact – to having felt received, heard and understood.

As the therapist strives to experience and offer empathic understanding, client change and growth may be fostered in many different ways. Reviewing a transcript of a half-hour therapy session conducted by Carl Rogers, Nat Raskin and Rogers identified several characteristics of Carl's communications:

> The interview exemplifies the therapeutic mechanism of empathy backed by genuineness and unconditional positive regard. It helps the client to (1) examine her problems in a way that shifts responsibility from others to herself, (2) experience emotions in the immediacy of the therapy encounter, (3) accept aspects of self formerly denied to awareness, and (4) raise her general level of self-regard.
>
> (Rogers and Raskin 1989: p. 178)

Carl's initial verbalisations were open. He did not try to reassure the client, ask questions or delve into their history, or take on the responsibility of providing a solution or focusing therapy (thereby living by his belief in the inner resources of clients). As a consequence of perceiving that she has been understood, the client broadens her view. Rather than talking *about* her emotions, she experiences them in the here and now. She moves towards talking about herself and away from narrative concerning others, and as a consequence of experiencing unconditional positive regard from Carl, she moves towards greater self-acceptance. Their relationship becomes more reciprocal.

What psychological purpose is served by attempting to duplicate, as it were, the perceptual field of the client in the mind of the counsellor? Clients experience therapists in a variety of ways, but some common threads do emerge. For one client:

> Notice how the significant theme of the relationship is, 'we were mostly *me* working together on my situation as I found it.' The two selves have somehow become one while remaining two – 'we were *me*.' This idea is repeated several times. . . . The impression is that the client was in one sense 'talking to herself', and yet that this was a very different process when she talked to herself through the medium of another person.
>
> (Rogers 1951: p. 39)

For another client:

> Perhaps it would be accurate to say that the attitudes which she could express but could not accept as a part of herself became acceptable when an alternate self, the counselor, looked upon them with acceptance . . .
>
> (Rogers 1951: p. 39)

We have already seen that *if* conducive therapeutic conditions prevail, *then* clients are more readily able to access their ('self-referent') psychological and physiological inner flow of experiencing. Indeed, you may even have reacted to the idea of a momentary pause in order to try it and experience it for yourself. Very often therapists are confident in their sensing of something difficult or even fearful going on within clients, yet feel less secure about the content and personal meanings embraced by the client's here-and-now experiencing. In order to perception check, the therapist might volunteer a *tentative* voicing of their empathic grasping, while being constantly alert and willing to move with the client's feelings and personal meanings that emerge as a consequence of the therapist *striving* to understand. Rogers wrote:

> Now here's what has interested me about this . . . it's always puzzled me. Some words fit what is being experienced and others do not. I've noticed that, in trying to check my understanding, I might say: 'Is it that you are so angry at your father?', 'No, that's not quite it.' 'Is it that you hate him?', 'No.' 'Is it that you feel contempt?', 'Yes! Contempt. That's what I feel.' That's the kind of response, as though at some level there is a verbal form which really fits what's being experienced. It's quite striking sometimes. I don't pretend to understand it, but it's

something that has intrigued me. How is it that, if he hadn't been able to describe his feelings, one word fits exactly and another word quite similar to it doesn't fit at all? Puzzling . . .

(Rogers and Teich 1992: pp. 62–3)

Especially when reflecting in retrospect upon their developmental movements over the course of a diploma in client-centred therapy, trainees have often related how at the beginning it felt safer to rely on implementing skills that they had learned or been taught than to venture into communicating empathic under-standing. The *fear* of owning that a perception might be inaccurate seemed to far outweigh the *embarrassment* of not quite getting a technique right. We have seen, too, that Rogers believed a further risk of the therapist experiencing and communicating empathy is that the *therapist* might change through the process as well as the client. Yet to understand another empathically is edifying in at least two fundamental respects:

I find when I am working with clients in distress, that to understand the bizarre world of a psychotic individual, or to understand and sense the attitudes of a person who feels that life is too tragic to bear, or to understand a man who feels that he is a worthless and inferior individual – each of these understandings somehow enriches me. I learn from these experiences in ways that change me, that make me a different and, I think, a more responsive person.

(Rogers 1961: pp. 18–19)

Thus counsellors themselves may be enriched through being this therapist core condition. However, even greater significance is the humbling privilege of being allowed to enter the private world of feelings and meanings – both 'courage and kindness and love and sensitivity' and terror, oddity, disillusionment and tragedy – and to be in awe of oneself and the other as this provision of understanding generates greater client self-understanding and self-acceptance. Being an active party in the change and growth of another is indeed an awesome, humbling privilege.

Empathy: Fay, an illustration

My genuine and respectful striving to empathically sense and understand Fay's world of feelings and meanings was central to the whole of our journey together. From moment to moment I would not only hang on her every word and expression, but also really try to sense what lay beneath or behind her commun-ications, and would tentatively venture what I believed I had gleaned. My own process was an internal seeking. What does this *shame*, for instance, actually *feel* like? What meanings are attached to feeling this way? As a consequence of seeking to sense such feelings and meanings, some empathic understanding was ventured, accompanied by a very close attendance to how Fay received my communications (verbally, paraverbally and non-verbally). I tried to follow her ongoing leads in every way.

Sometimes my sensing was very accurate, and that felt *good* to Fay – to feel honestly accepted and understood. At other times, I was a little off-beam – and that felt good to Fay, too, for in clarifying for me (which she willingly did), things crystallised for her as well. As we moved towards ending, she was able to say:

> I was a person who allowed myself to be exploited, and now I can see why. I feel warmth toward that me now, rather than despising and loathing myself. I do regret what happened, yet I am different now. I still feel very lonely, but I do not miss him: I miss some aspects of togetherness that being in a relationship can bring. I realise, in fact, that I do not miss him at all – rather, I miss the hopes and dreams, the potential that I initially saw in that relationship. I do not hate him anymore; I feel a little pitying of him (and pity doesn't feel too good, maybe I still need to work on that). I realise that at times I sensed his vulnerable inner self, and it was *that* part of him that I held out hope for. I have moved on now . . . It feels like I am a new, more real, me.

Client do

When asked what he was working towards as a therapist, Carl Rogers said:

> For myself, I have a rather simple definition, yet one which I think has a good many implications. I feel that I'm quite pleased in my work as a therapist if I find that my client and I, too, are – if we are both moving toward what I think of as greater openness to experience.
>
> (Rogers 1989: p. 75)

Client movement towards greater openness to experience is enabled through clients becoming better able to listen to and participate fully in their inner communications, and hence becoming more perceptive about themselves, others and the worlds that they inhabit. This *process of becoming* could hardly be described as static, and Rogers said that he felt rewarded when this process gets under way. The client also becomes more realistic and socialised:

> simply because one of the elements which he can't help but actualize in himself is the need and desire for closer human relationships; so for me, this concept of openness to experience describes a good deal of what I would hope to see in the more optimal person . . .
>
> (Rogers 1989: p. 75)

We have seen that client-centred therapy can be formulated as if (A) *then* (B), if (B) *then* (C), where (A) is a relationship founded on contact between an incongruent (vulnerable, anxious and defensive) client and an authentic, respectful and understanding therapist, and in which the client at least to some degree perceives that respectful empathy. (B) can represent the capacity and potential of clients, which is released as a consequence of being in (A). What is the outcome of (A) plus (B), (C)? Put simply, if the therapist can *be* the core conditions, what do clients *do*? In essence, client potential for self-actualising that is in harmony with the organism as a whole can be released and realised:

> The individual will reorganize himself at both the conscious and deeper levels of his personality in such a manner as to cope with life

more constructively, more intelligently, and in a more socialized as
well as a more satisfying way.

(Rogers 1961: p. 36)

Carl Rogers was able to base his comments on solid research findings, and could
state that even *limited* client experience of client-centred therapy would produce
changes in personality (attitudes and behaviour) that were both significant and
profound. The outcome is a more integrated and effective individual. So it had
been discovered that even relatively minimal engagement with client-centred
therapy results in fewer symptoms of what might, in other approaches to helping,
be labelled as 'neurosis', 'psychosis' or other 'personality problems' of some
description. Client-centred therapy results in clients moving towards having a
more realistic perception of the self. They become more like their ideal selves,
self-valuing increases, they exhibit higher levels of confidence and greater
autonomy, there is improved self-understanding, they become more open to
experiencing (that is, there is a marked decrease in denial and distortion), and
they become more accepting of the sovereignty and humanity of others.
Furthermore, there are behavioural changes as a result of psychological
growth. Clients become less frustrated by and recover more quickly from stress,
they are more mature and less defensive, and they are more flexible and creative.
As Rogers stated:

there can no longer be any doubt as to the effectiveness of such a
relationship in producing personality change.

(Rogers 1961: p. 36)

One client said 'Now that I see all that, I guess it's really up to me', and Carl
Rogers said:

I think as the person becomes aware of these various factors in his
background, he can make realistic and sensible choices as to how he's
going to both live with and transcend the circumstances of the past . . .
I don't believe in free will in the sense that a person's free to do
anything, but to deny the reality of the significance of choice as the
strict behaviorists do is totally unrealistic . . . the person can and does
choose significantly. I've always been rather pleased that our research-
ers in psychotherapy have shown that the element that probably
changes most in individual therapy is the person's concept of himself.
He moves toward being a more confident self, more acceptant of
himself; self-hatred decreases. As a person feels genuinely confident
of who he is and what he's capable of doing, he goes ahead to utilize
his past, his conditioning, and the biological basis of his being in more
constructive ways.

(Rogers and Evans 1975: pp. 76–7)

Both at the time but even more so in retrospect, Rogers realised the importance of
research into 'delinquents' undertaken by Bill Kell, through which it was
discovered (much to the astonishment of the research team) that in terms of
predicting future behaviour, self-understanding *far* outweighed such factors as
family environment and other social and economic concerns:

Actually, it was so shocking to us at the time of the original study – this was many years ago – that we frankly didn't believe the findings.

(Rogers and Evans 1975: pp. 77–9)

As a result of this scepticism, Helen McNeil replicated the research, and again self-understanding proved to be the most significant factor. Yet again the research team could hardly believe these findings, and so embarked on a sub-analysis, about which Rogers wrote:

Again, self-understanding . . . correlated more highly with their behavior. So the essence of that seemed to be that the person who is realistic about himself, who has a pretty good comprehension of what he's up against, and what factors have influenced his behavior, has a much better chance of controlling his behavior. He can make choices. At the time I didn't appreciate the full depth of that study. It's taken a good many years for me to realize that our findings were more significant than I thought at the time.

(Rogers and Evans 1975: pp. 77–9)

So if a fundamental aspect of client-centred therapy is increasing awareness, acceptance and reorganising of the self, here was evidence from 'beyond' therapy that corroborated the social significance of this.

In expressing a real trust in the potential (the actualising tendency) that resides in all of us, Rogers said:

it seems to me that you could speak of the goal toward which therapy moves, and I guess the goal toward which maturity moves in an individual, as being *becoming*, or being knowingly and acceptingly that which one most deeply is.

(Rogers 1989: p. 62)

The client-centred therapist is committed to an ongoing, moment-by-moment striving to authentically and respectfully empathise with clients. How might clients experience this?

the concentrated attentiveness to his person, concerns, and his feelings is an extraordinary event in the client's life, naturally increasing his sense of substantiality and reality and lending dignity to his self and his concerns.

(Barton 1974: p. 192)

From first contact onwards, clients ideally experience both a meaningful and an acceptant connection and feel fully received for whoever and however they are. All disclosures are met with respect and an attempt at understanding, rather than being contemptuously dismissed as 'silly', as is so often the case with both their own inner and external communications. As self-expression meets with an authentic, acceptant empathy, so clients feel increasingly safe in further verbalising what is going on for them, and they gradually begin to incorporate previously denied or distorted experiencing into their self concepts. This in turn influences their behaviour (actions or inaction):

> As I listened to therapeutic interviews . . . I realized that when a person is functioning well and has profited a lot from therapy, you find they're open to their experience. They're able to express what they're feeling – what they're experiencing – and to assimilate that into their concept of themselves and guide their behavior in terms of it.
>
> (Rogers and Russell 2002: pp. 256–7)

As therapy progresses, clients gradually adopt a client-centred way of being *towards themselves*. In a sense, the *process* of client-centred therapy could almost be represented by the therapist 'core' conditions in reverse – that is, a congruent therapist experiences unconditional positive regard towards and strives to empathically understand an incongruent client. As a consequence of perceiving these conditions from the therapist, clients move towards experiencing greater self-acceptance (especially as a consequence of feeling respected by a significant other) and deeper self-understanding (especially as a consequence of being reciprocally involved in a process of genuine empathic striving). As a consequence of greater self-acceptance and self-understanding, more and more experience becomes available to awareness, and hence may become integrated aspects of the client's concept of self:

> The self is now more congruent with the experiencing. Thus, the persons have become, in their attitudes toward themselves, more caring and acceptant, more empathic and understanding, more real and congruent. But these three elements are the very ones that both experience and research indicate are the attitudes of an effective therapist. So we are perhaps not overstating the total picture if we say that an empathic understanding by another enables a person to become a more effective growth enhancer, a more effective therapist, for himself or herself.
>
> (Rogers 1980: p. 159)

No surrender!

We have seen that upon entering therapy clients are likely to be vulnerable, anxious and tense as a consequence of their defensive psychological denial and distortion processes no longer being able to entirely prevent *some* awareness of their incongruence. Conversely:

> We may say that freedom from inner tension, or psychological adjustment, exists when the concept of self is at least roughly congruent with all the experiences of the organism.
>
> (Rogers 1951: p. 513)

Rogers gave the example of a woman who denied her sexual impulses (this was in the 1950s) because she believed them to be taboo, or improper, or immoral. Therefore they *had* to be denied because they simply could not coexist with her view of herself as she *should* be, namely 'proper' and moral. Many of her *shoulds* and *oughts* were values introjected both from significant others and from her society. However, as therapy progresses the client is able to accept and understand both of these facets of herself. She can accept her sexual desires as 'normal' *and* respect and understand cultural moral values as being significant in her world.

She can more fully *be* herself rather than being in conflict, strenuously striving to achieve victory for one aspect of herself over another – even though neither facet of herself is overly willing to surrender or accept defeat:

> The feeling of reduction of inner tension is something that clients experience as they make progress in 'being the real me' or in developing 'a new feeling about myself' . . . The cost of maintaining an alertness of defense to prevent various experiences from being symbolized in consciousness is obviously great.
>
> (Rogers 1951: p. 513)

In a medical practice, many patients are referred to counselling because either they have told their doctor, or their doctor has told them, that they are *depressed*. These clients often arrive at their first therapy session already having been prescribed antidepressant medication. Thus there is a very powerful underlying value that the patient *should not* be depressed. Usually the patients themselves feel that there is something wrong with them (which is why they went to see their GP in the first place), and this is confirmed by their having been prescribed medication that is intended to 'help them get better' or 'recover' from their depression.

Yet, more often than not, there really would be something odd or weird about these clients if they did *not* feel depressed. As human beings who have experienced or are experiencing difficult or tragic circumstances, *of course* they feel low. When these clients experience authentic unconditional positive regard and empathic understanding from their counsellor, they begin to realise that they are not 'abnormal' after all – being received as human beings who are worthy of respect *as and how they are* means that they can begin to accept themselves as and how they are. Furthermore, the feelings, thoughts and behaviours that they believe they should not have or ought not to have begin to seem understandable and therefore normal, acceptable and real consequences of living – they begin to reconnect with humanity. 'Depressed' clients very often describe their feeling of exhaustion – even getting up in the morning just feels like too much trouble, and the effort involved in getting through another day just doesn't feel worthwhile. Yet very often it seems that a huge portion of the inner energy available to them has been spent in fighting and trying to vanquish their sinister, bizarre, unacceptable feelings and thoughts. Their inner experience is of wanting to stay curled up in bed feeling miserable and alone, but there is an internal voice saying 'pull yourself together, stop being a self-indulgent wimp, and get on with life – there are many people worse off than you!'. Other internal dialogues might be characterised by, on the one hand, feeling insignificant and worthless while, on the other hand, there is a wailing, plaintive 'What about me?'. Many thoughts or wishes might be dismissed as silly, irrational or needless. All in all, a massive amount of energy is expended in striving to resolve this exhausting inner battle that rages on – no wonder that there is a reluctance to emerge from the cocoon of sleep, or a yearning to sleep for ever. Yet when clients begin to *be* their depression rather than fighting it, there is a huge metaphorical 'inner sigh' as the client relaxes into a greater acceptance of their wholeness, and gradually the vast stores of energy used up in a conflict that *inevitably* tends towards there being winners and losers, victors and vanquished, can gradually be recouped or recharged and redirected towards the more constructive tendencies in all of us. As more experiencing becomes available to consciousness, the client can move towards celebrating the diversity of all of their selves, rather than striving to impose a harsh regime in which some selves have to surrender while others bask in their tyrannical glory:

> The term 'available to consciousness' . . . is deliberately chosen. It is the fact that all experiences, impulses, sensations are *available* that is important, and not necessarily the fact that they are present in consciousness. It is the organization of the concept of self *against* the symbolization of certain experiences contradictory to itself, which is the significant negative fact. Actually, when all experiences are assimilated in relationship to the self and made a part of the structure of the self, there tends to be *less* of what is called 'self-consciousness' on the part of the individual. Behavior becomes more spontaneous, expression of attitudes is less guarded, because the self can accept such attitudes and such behavior as a part of itself. Frequently a client at the beginning of therapy expresses real fear that others might discover his real self. 'As soon as I start thinking about what *I* am, I have such a terrible conflict at what I am that it makes me feel awful. It's such a self-depreciation that I hope nobody ever knows it . . . I'm afraid to act natural, I guess, because I just don't feel as though I like myself.' In this frame of mind, behavior must always be guarded, cautious, self-conscious. But when this same client has come to accept deeply the fact that 'I am what I am', then she can be spontaneous and can lose her self-consciousness.
>
> (Rogers 1951: p. 515)

From four to one against to two to one on!

As a consequence of experiencing the therapist conditions and of feeling received, there is less potential for clients to experience tension or anxiety, and so they become less vulnerable. Due to there being a reduced possibility of threat to the self-concept, the self-concepts of clients change, as they are able to assimilate previously denied or distorted experiencing. The self-concept has become more flexible and inclusive, and the client has moved away from feeling unworthy of respect (a feeling that was based largely on standards introjected from others) and towards greater self-acceptance. There is less and less need for defensiveness as each new disclosure meets with therapist respect and understanding and, more importantly, self-respect and self-understanding:

> One study showed that at the beginning of therapy, current attitudes toward self were four to one negative, but in the final fifth of therapy self-attitudes were twice as often positive as negative.
>
> (Rogers 1961: p. 65)

Clients become more self-directing as both they and their therapists trust in the wisdom of the whole organism – the client's internal locus of evaluation. Reduced defensiveness (due to the absence of threat from both the client's own self-concept and an acceptant, understanding therapist) leads to clients becoming more adaptable, as their behaviour becomes increasingly based on more accurate and complete data (as less and less is denied or distorted) – the facts are always friendly! Clients become more open to their full experiencing, and the *ideal* self changes, too, becoming more realistic and therefore the person's aims are more achievable. The chasm between clients as they want to be and clients as they are is greatly diminished, which means that they are less and less likely to have 'out-of-character' experiences – and this feeling of enhanced self-control in turn leads to yet greater self-acceptance:

> More of the total experience of the organism is directly incorporated into the self; or more accurately, the self tends to be discovered in the total experience of the organism. The client feels he is his 'real' self, his organic self.
>
> (Rogers 1951: pp. 531–2)

As a consequence, tension of *all* types (physiological as well as psychological) continues to decrease as each new step on this journey of personal development continues to meet with unconditional prizing and empathy – from the therapist and, increasingly, internal acceptance and understanding. As a consequence of feeling yet further self-acceptance, clients become more accepting of others (and the ideals that they project on to others also become more realistic and therefore achievable). In large part due to the reduced need to protect their own concepts of self, others are now perceived as unique and separate individuals, worthy of their own dignity:

> The best definition of what constitutes integration appears to be this statement that all the sensory and visceral experiences are admissible to awareness through accurate symbolization, and organizable into one system which is internally consistent and which is, or is related to, the structure of self. Once this type of integration occurs, then the tendency toward growth can become fully operative, and the individual moves in the directions normal to all organic life. When the self-structure is able to accept and take account in consciousness of the organic experiences, when the organizational system is expansive enough to contain them, then clear integration and a sense of direction are achieved, and the individual feels that his strength can be and is directed toward the clear purpose of actualization and enhancement of a unified organism.
>
> (Rogers 1951: pp. 513–14)

The client rejects the desire to control or manipulate others, preferring instead to *be* the greater valuing and enrichment that increased awareness of self and others brings. The 'fully functioning person' is able both to accurately perceive and to assimilate and integrate all relevant experiencing:

> If I feel hatred, I can assimilate the fact that I'm a hating person; I hate this individual. If I feel love, I'm able to recognize that that's what I'm feeling. If I'm frightened, the same, so that when one is really open to all of the experiences going on in the organism, one is a fully functioning person.
>
> (Rogers and Russell 2002: p. 252)

Being fully functioning – open to a multiplicity of experiences – involves a readiness to engage with both here-and-now factors (such as social and cultural expectations, satisfactory and unsatisfactory relationships with others, physical requirements, legal demands, and so on) and the personal feelings and meanings that have grown out of the past. Every new stimulus is evaluated in terms of the whole person, which means that the actualising tendency and self-actualising are now harnessed together rather than being in conflict.

Rogers wrote that the valuing process which resides in the 'fully functioning' or 'psychologically mature' person is the most sensitive such process that exists in the entire universe as we know it. He was also keen to point out that although this valuing process does operate on whether or not experiencing maintains and enhances (self-)actualisation, it is nevertheless *not selfish*, because the fundamental nature of human beings is highly *social* (see, for instance, Rogers 1989: pp. 137–8). Nor are fully functioning individuals entirely 'perfect' – we have already learned that Rogers saw the human being not as seeking stasis only, and that openness to experience and self-acceptance includes being non-defensive about failings and negative feelings as well as positive qualities:

> This emerging person would not bring utopia. He would make mistakes, be partially corrupted, go overboard in certain directions.
> (Rogers and Evans 1975: pp. 173–4)

However, the 'person of tomorrow' – the fully functioning, psychologically mature person – would tend to live in (or create) a culture (and subcultures) within which certain values, beliefs and attitudes have significant emphasis. Non-defensive openness to self and experience would apply in all relationships (with partners, family and at work, for instance), and the 'style' of interpersonal relationships would be more deeply rooted in the principles of the person-centred approach. There would be greater respect for the dignity of all people, irrespective of such issues as social status, gender, ethnicity, or perceived and real disadvantages. Groupings of people (in communities, at work, in education, and so on) would be less gargantuan and impersonal, and greater respect towards and reciprocity with nature would feature. Resources of all kinds would be shared with greater equity, and there would be less materialism for its own sake, and less greed. There would be reduced authoritarianism and bureaucracy, with sensitivity to human needs outweighing administrative and control needs, and leadership would become less significant. Concern for those who would benefit from assistance would be genuine and caring, and scientific creativity would become more humane, too. Indeed, there would be greater creativity of all kinds in all areas. The human being has moved:

> toward the exploration of self and the development of the richness of the total, individual, responsible human soma – mind and body.
> (Rogers and Evans 1975: pp. 173–4)

Thus in becoming more open to self and others, in becoming more aware of self and others, in becoming more acceptant of self and others, and in becoming more understanding of self and others, people become more able to live their lives meaningfully, more:

> able to love; able to receive love.
> (Rogers and Russell 2002: p. 258)

Afterwords

> Our civilization does not yet have enough faith in the social sciences to utilize their findings.
>
> (Rogers 1961: p. 335)

We have found that if a therapist can initiate a helping relationship with an incongruent person, founded on the therapist experiencing authentic unconditional positive regard and empathic understanding and the client perceiving these therapist qualities, then this is all that is necessary and sufficient for people to change and grow. Have faith! Trust in the resources and capacities of clients! As Rogers said:

> I'm pretty good at living and letting live, so the fact that people have held different points of view from mine has never troubled me much. Criticisms that come from honest viewpoints which differ quite sharply from mine are OK with me. I suppose the kind of criticism that I've liked least is the notion, which used to be expressed in many ways over the course of years, that the client-centered approach was a pretty shallow approach. It might do for dealing with superficial problems, but it really had not much to do with the deeper problems of personality. That is just not true. This criticism has probably troubled me more than any other I can think of, because I don't think I am superficial. You can't do anything but laugh off the fact that a lot of criticism is based on a complete lack of understanding of what I've been doing and what my associates have been doing.
>
> (Rogers and Evans 1975: p. 114)

The would-be therapist is faced with a choice – either we can utilise what we know to control, manipulate, teach and, effectively, depersonalise and enslave people (often without their knowing) into becoming what we or society wish them to be, or we can opt for freedom, to provide conditions that are conducive to growth, creativity and autonomy (whether it be for individuals or groups of people):

> There are really only a few psychologists who have contributed ideas that help to set people free, making them psychologically free and self-responsible, encouraging them in decision making and problem solving.
>
> (Rogers and Evans 1975: pp. 65–6)

Rogers stated that he was particularly disappointed in academic psychologists working within the 'great' learning establishments, and conceded that he:

> had very little influence on academic psychology, in the lecture hall, the textbook, or the laboratory. There is some passing mention of my thinking, my theories, or my approach to therapy, but, by and large,

> I think I have been a painfully embarrassing phenomenon to the academic psychologist. *I do not fit*. Increasingly I have come to agree with that assessment.
>
> (Rogers and Evans 1975: p. 126)

Rogers nevertheless maintained that *of course* we need to remain sceptical, to continually engage in research and question our findings, theories and practices – yet in doing so we can remain committed to the sovereignty of the person. As Carl said (in response to Richard Evans):

> And I like your word, *commitment*, because I think that's probably better than my use of *belief* or *conviction*.
>
> (Rogers and Evans 1975: p. 69)

Indeed, when asked to state who had most shaped his work, Carl had no hesitation in saying that it was his clients, and that he had paid attention to their 'raw data' that emerged from the tape recording of sessions and the subsequent reflection upon the experiencing:

> I feel that almost everything I've learned about personality, about interpersonal relationships, about personality dynamics came not from books or from some charismatic teacher, but from direct experience with the people I've been working with . . . I guess something I take some pride in is that I always wanted to get close to the raw data.
>
> (Rogers and Evans 1975: p. 109 and pp. 112–13)

So what of the future? Of his own developmental trends, Rogers said:

> I will introduce quite a personal note here. I find I'm not much good at planning my future. I *ooze* toward my future. That is one term I like to use because it reminds me of an amoeba that sends out these protoplasmic tentacles and then if it runs into something aversive, it draws back, but it flows in the direction that seems rewarding. And I feel that's the nature of my professional life.
>
> (Rogers and Evans 1975: p. 117)

Of the world, Rogers acknowledged that evidence of negativity is all around us, yet he remained optimistic:

> To me, the person who offers the most hope in our crazy world today, which could be wiping itself out, is the individual who is most fully aware – most fully aware of what is going on within himself: physiologically, feeling-wise, his thoughts; also aware of the external world that is impinging on him. The more fully he is aware of the whole system, or perhaps context – the more hope there is that he would live a balanced human life without the violence, the craziness, the deceit, the horrible things that we tend to do to each other in the modern world.
>
> (Rogers 1989: pp. 188–9)

And what of the future of client-centred therapy? We face threats from without – those who ignore the evidence of research that sometimes they themselves have sponsored, evidence which time and time again demonstrates that what is most helpful is a therapeutic relationship founded on authentic respect and under-standing. We face threats from within – those who lack the discipline of Rogers and view congruence as meaning that anything goes, agencies responsible for the validation of training (governmental and academic) who reduce an exquisite intimacy to the mechanical implementation of skills, and those who lack the courage or support to hold on to the therapist conditions as both necessary and sufficient. Yet just as the client-centred therapist trusts in the capacity of clients, maybe we need to trust in our own resources, too:

> I hope you would find it possible to trust your deepest self. I think that the follies and tragedies of the world result from people being fearful of themselves, not knowing themselves, and certainly being unwilling to trust the deepest level of selfhood.
>
> (Rogers 1989: pp. 197–8)

There *is* hope.

I simply say with all my heart:

Power to the emerging person and the revolution he carries within.
(Rogers and Evans 1975: p. 175)

Emerge!

Why be the magician when you can be the magic?

Bibliography

Barrett-Lennard G (1959) *Dimensions of the client's experience of his therapist associated with personality change*. Unpublished doctoral dissertation, University of Chicago, Chicago.

Barton A (1974) *Three Worlds of Therapy*. Mayfield Publishing Company, Palo Alto, CA.

Bergin A and Jasper L (1969) Correlates of empathy in psychotherapy: a replication. *J Abnorm Psychol*. 74: 477–81.

Bergin A and Solomon S (1970) Personality and performance correlates of empathic understanding in psychotherapy. In: J Hart and T Tomlinson (eds) *New Directions in Client-Centered Therapy*. Houghton Mifflin, Boston, MA.

Bergman DV (1951) Counseling method and client responses. *J Consult Psychol*. 15: 216–44.

Berwick K and Rogers C (1983) *Carl Rogers Counsels Keith Berwick*. CSP/CCTPCAS video.*

Budman SH and Gurman AS (1988) *Theory and Practice of Brief Therapy*. Guilford Press, New York.

Farber B, Brink D and Raskin P (eds) (1996) *The Psychotherapy of Carl Rogers*. Guilford Press, New York.

Farson R (1955) *Introjection in the psychotherapeutic relationship*. Unpublished doctoral dissertation, University of Chicago, Chicago.

Fiedler FE (1953) Quantitative studies on the role of therapists' feelings toward their patients. In OH Mowrer (ed.) *Psychotherapy Theory and Research*. Ronald Press, New York.

Frick W (1989) *Humanistic Psychology: conversations with Maslow, Murphy, Rogers*. Wyndham Hall Press, Bristol. This includes a conversation with Carl Rogers (1969).

Friedli K, King M, Lloyd M and Horder J (1997) Randomised controlled assessment of non-directive psychotherapy versus routine general practitioner care. *Lancet*. 350: 1662–5.

Greenfield S (2000) *Brain Story*. BBC books, London.

Hampshire Association for Counselling (2001) *Counsellor Resources Directory*. Hampshire Association for Counselling.

Kelly G (1955) *The Psychology of Personal Constructs*. Norton, New York.

King M, Sibbald B, Ward E *et al.* (2000). Randomised controlled trial of non-directive counselling, cognitive behaviour therapy and usual general practitioner care in the management of depression as well as mixed anxiety and depression in primary care. *BMJ*. 321: 1389–92.

Kirschenbaum H (1979) *On Becoming Carl Rogers*. Delacorte Press, New York.

Laing RD (1965) *The Divided Self*. Pelican, Middlesex, UK.

McLeary RA and Lazarus RS (1949) Autonomic discrimination without awareness. *J Pers*. 18: 171–9.

Mearns D (2002) *Developing Person-Centred Counselling*. Sage Publications, London.

Mellor-Clark J, Connell J, Barkham M and Cummins P (2001) Counselling outcomes in primary health care: a CORE system data profile. *Eur J Psychother Counsell Health*. 4: 65–86.

Nelson-Jones R and Patterson CH (1975) Measuring client-centred attitudes. *Br J Guidance Counsell*. 3: 228–36.

Patterson CH (2000) *Understanding Psychotherapy: fifty years of client-centred theory and practice*. PCCS Books.

Patterson CH and Watkins CE Jnr (1996) *Theories of Psychotherapy*. HarperCollins College Publishers, New York.

Prouty G, van Werde G and Portner M (2002) *Pre-Therapy*. PCCS Books, Llangarron, Ross-on-Wye.

Rogers C (1937) The clinical psychologist's approach to personality problems. *Family.* **18:** 233–43.

Rogers C (1939) *Clinical Treatment of the Problem Child.* Houghton Mifflin, Riverside Press, Cambridge, MA.

Rogers C (1942) *Counseling and Psychotherapy.* Houghton Mifflin, Boston, New York.

Rogers C (1946) Significant aspects of client-centered therapy. *Am Psychol.* **1:** 415–22.

Rogers C (1951) *Client-Centered Therapy.* Constable, London.

Rogers C (1957a) The necessary and sufficient conditions of therapeutic personality change. *J Consult Psychol.* **21:** 95–103.

Rogers C (1957b) A therapist's view of the good life. *Humanist.* **17:** 299–300.

Rogers C (1959) A theory of therapy, personality, and interpersonal relationships, as developed in the client-centered framework. In: S Koch (ed.) *Psychology: a study of a science. Study 1. Volume 3. Formulations of the person and the social context.* McGraw-Hill, New York, Toronto, London.*

Rogers C (1961) *On Becoming a Person.* Constable, London.

Rogers C (ed.) (1967) *The Therapeutic Relationship and its Impact: a study of psychotherapy with schizophrenics.* The University of Wisconsin Press, Madison, Milwaukee and London.

Rogers C (1975) Empathic: an unappreciated way of being. *Counsel Psychol.* **5:** 2–10.

Rogers C (1978) *Carl Rogers on Personal Power.* Constable, London.

Rogers C (1980) *A Way of Being.* Houghton Mifflin, Boston, New York.

Rogers C (1981) Notes on Rollo May. In: H Kirschenbaum and V Land Henderson (1989) *Carl Rogers: Dialogues.* Houghton-Mifflin, Boston.

Rogers C (1985) *Personally Speaking: Carl Rogers.* John Masterson interview, RTE Dublin television programme, recorded on 23 November 1985.*

Rogers C (1986) *Politics and Innocence: a humanistic debate.* Saybrook, Dallas, Texas.

Rogers C (1987a) Client-centered? Person-centered? *Person-Centered Rev.* **2:** 11–13.

Rogers C (1987b) What areas of person-centred theory or practice require further research? **2:** 252.

Rogers C (1989) *Carl Rogers: dialogues* (H Kirschenbaum and V Land Henderson, eds). Houghton Mifflin, Boston.

Rogers C and Buber M (1957) In: H Kirschenbaum and V Land Henderson (1989) *Carl Rogers: Dialogues.* Houghton Mifflin, Boston.

Rogers C and Frick W (1967) Conversation with Carl. In: *Humanistic Psychology: conversations with Maslow, Murphy, Rogers.* Wyndham Hall Press, Bristol, Indiana.

Rogers C and Stevens B (1967) *Person to Person: the problem of being human.* Souvenir Press, Guernsey, Channel Islands.

Rogers C and Truax C (1967) The therapeutic conditions antecedent to change: a theoretical view. In: C Rogers, E Gendlin, D Kiesler and C Truax (eds) *The Therapeutic Relationship with Schizophrenics.* Wisconsin Press, Madison, WI.

Rogers C and Evans R (1975) *Carl Rogers: the man and his ideas.* EP Dutton, New York.

Rogers C and Evans R (1981) *In Dialogue with Carl Rogers.* Praeger, New York.

Rogers C and Ryback D (1984) One alternative to nuclear planetary suicide. *Counsel Psychol.* **12:** 3–12.

Rogers C and Barfield GS (1985) *Empathy: an exploration.* Center for Studies of the Person video.*

Rogers C and Sanford R (1985) *In Conversation.* Center for Studies of the Person video.*

Rogers C and Raskin N (1989) Person-centred therapy. In: R Corsini and D Wedding (eds) *Current Psychotherapies.* Peacock, Itasca, Illinois.

Rogers C and Teich N (1992) Conversation with Carl Rogers (1985). In: N Teich (ed.) *Rogerian Perspectives: collaborative rhetoric for oral and written communication.* Ablex Publishing Corporation, Norwood, New Jersey.

Rogers C and Russell D (2002) *Carl Rogers: the quiet revolutionary.* Penmarin Books, Roseville, CA.

Rogers C, Kohut H and Erickson M (1986) A personal perspective on some similarities and differences. *Person-Centered Rev.* **1**: 125–40.

Rogers N (1997) Counselling and creativity: an interview with Natalie Rogers. *Br J Guidance Counsell.* **25**: 263–73.

Seeman J (1949) A study of the process of nondirective therapy. *J Consult Psychol.* **13**: 157–67.

Shlien J (1986) In: *Reflection of Feelings* by Carl Rogers. *Person-Centered Rev.* **1**: 375–7.

Slack S (1985) Reflections on a workshop with Carl Rogers. *J Human Psychol.* **25**: 35–42.

Snyder WU (1943) An investigation of the nature of non-directive psychotherapy, PhD thesis, Ohio State University, Ohio.

Standal S (1954) *The need for positive regard: a contribution to client-centered theory.* Unpublished doctoral dissertation. University of Chicago, Chicago.*

Tolman M (1990) *Single Session Therapy: maximizing the effect of the first (and often only) therapeutic encounter.* Jossey-Bass, San Francisco.

Vincent S (1998) *PC or Not PC . . . that is the question.* BAPCA AGM address, 14 March 1998.*

Vincent S (1999a) *On becoming person-centred?* Masters dissertation, University of East Anglia, Norwich.*

Vincent S (1999b) On becoming more whole? Necking in Glasgow. *Person-Centred Pract.* **7**: 95–101.

Vincent S (1999c) *A Training Trip Through Empathy.* CCTPCAS publication.*

Vincent S (2000a) From Whole to Hole to Whole. In: *Person-To-Person*, BAPCA Newsletter.* pp. 8–10.

Vincent S (2000b) *Failing or Fortunate? Striving for revising.* CCTPCAS publication.*

Vincent S (2001) Setting Aside or Erupting? *Person-Centred Pract.* **9**: 97–104.

Vincent S (2002a) Client-centred therapy: conditions, process and theory. *Person-Centred Pract.* **10**: 35–44.

Vincent S (2002b) *Empathy: an inter-view.* CCTPCAS publication.*

Vincent S (2002c) *Evaluating Empathy?* CCTPCAS publication.*

Vincent S (2004) Approach and outcomes. In: *Southampton Primary Care Counselling Services Summary Report 2004.** Southampton Primary Care Counselling Service.

Index

Printed and bound by CPI Group (UK) Ltd, Croydon, CR0 4YY

23/10/2024

01777678-0004